NEUROPLASTICITY FOR BEGINNERS

HOW TO BOOST BRAIN COGNITION, BRAIN HEALTH, AND IMPROVE MEMORY TO SLOW DOWN AGE-RELATED COGNITIVE DECLINE

HECTOR J BORDAS

To my son Andrew…

CONTENTS

INTRODUCTION

About a year ago, I met a man named David who had almost given up hope. After struggling with memory loss and cognitive decline, he felt trapped in a fog — until something remarkable happened. Through deliberate practices designed to engage his brain, David experienced a profound transformation. His memory improved, and his thinking became clearer. His life changed in ways he had never imagined possible. This change was not due to some miracle drug or high-tech gadget. It was the power of neuroplasticity at work.

Neuroplasticity is the brain's ability to change and adapt. The brain can rewire itself in response to new experiences, learning, and even injury. This concept may sound complex, but it is simple at its core. Neuroplasticity is like a muscle that gets stronger with use. Just as we can train our bodies to be fit and strong, we can train our brains to be more agile and resilient.

My journey with neuroplasticity began by witnessing the cognitive decline of my parents, which ultimately resulted in dementia, the passing of my father, and the mental decline of my mother. I had to find tools, techniques, practices, and anything that would help prevent or, at the very least, minimize a similar situation happening to me.

I was unfamiliar with neuroplasticity and skeptical of its ability to rewire our brains. Although I had always been curious about how the brain works, the idea that we could change its structure seemed far-fetched.

However, I became convinced when I saw evidence in scientific studies and real-life examples. During my research and personal exploration of the topic, I discovered the incredible potential that lies within our brains.

This realization compelled me to share this knowledge with others and tell them about the human brain's untapped potential. My goal is to provide you with the knowledge and tools to harness the power of neuroplasticity. This book is about more than just understanding the science; it is about applying it to improve your life.

Nurturing and enhancing neuroplasticity is something we can do during our everyday routines. We, as humans, often need to pay more attention to our ability to grow, learn, and adapt. This book will show you how to incorporate practices that promote brain health and cognitive function. It is a hands-on guide designed to help you enhance your quality of life. You will find practical strategies that you can start implementing today.

Since this book is a guide to understanding and leveraging neuroplasticity, its objectives are as follows. First, I want to demystify neuroplasticity and make it accessible to everyone. Second, I will provide practical applications that you can use to improve your brain health. Lastly, I will share success stories, like David's, to illustrate the transformative power of these practices.

Each chapter of this book focuses on different aspects of neuroplasticity. You will learn about the science behind it and delve into practical exercises and real-life examples. We will explore habits, types of exercises, nutrition, supplements, and meditation. Each chapter builds on the previous one, providing a comprehensive approach to enhancing neuroplasticity.

Some practical applications include simple habits like learning a new skill, engaging in physical exercise, and practicing mindfulness. You will also discover how certain foods and supplements can support brain health.

As you read this book, please take some time to reflect on your mental habits and health and consider how to apply these principles to unlock your brain's potential. The journey of personal growth and cognitive enhancement is within your reach. All it takes is an open mind and a willingness to experiment with the strategies outlined within this book.

Understanding and applying the principles of neuroplasticity can transform your life. Although it is based on scientific research, it is written for everyone. You will find valuable insights and practical advice if you are new to this concept or already familiar with it.

Come with me on this journey to discover the power of neuroplasticity and how it can enhance our lives. The potential for growth and change is limitless, and your adventure begins now!

CHAPTER ONE
UNDERSTANDING NEUROPLASTICITY

Maria, an older woman, suffered a severe stroke that left her unable to speak or move her right side. Doctors warned her family that her recovery would be minimal, if at all. Yet, against all odds, Maria's determination and targeted neurological exercises led to a remarkable recovery. She regained her speech and mobility and even took up painting—a passion she never had before. This incredible transformation wasn't due to some miracle cure but was a testament to the power of neuroplasticity. Neuroplasticity is not just a scientific term; it's a profound force that can reshape lives.

1.1 WHAT IS NEUROPLASTICITY? AN INTRODUCTORY GUIDE

Neuroplasticity is the brain's ability to reorganize itself by forming new neural connections throughout life. In simpler terms, your brain is not set in stone. It can change, adapt, and grow, even as you age. Think of neuroplasticity as the brain's way of staying flexible and resilient, continually updating its wiring in response to new experiences, learning, and even injury. This level of adaptability allows us to learn new skills, recover from brain injuries, and adapt to new situations.

The fundamental principles of neuroplasticity revolve around the brain's capacity to change in response to experience, environment, and even injury. When you learn a new skill, your brain creates and strengthens pathways to make that skill easier to perform. Conversely, those pathways can weaken if you stop using a particular skill. This principle is often described as "use it or lose it." For example, when you play a musical instrument, the brain areas responsible for hand coordination and auditory processing become more active and develop stronger connections. If you stop practicing, those connections may weaken, but the potential for reactivation remains.

Neuroplasticity is not just a theoretical concept; it's a crucial part of everyday life. Think about the simple act of learning a new language. Your brain creates new neural pathways to help you remember vocabulary and understand grammar as you practice. The more you practice, the stronger these pathways become, making recalling and using the language much easier. Similarly, when you take up a new hobby like painting or sewing, your brain undergoes structural changes to accommodate these new skills. These changes are not just superficial; they involve the growth of new neurons and strengthening synaptic connections, fundamentally altering your brain's structure and function.

Historically, the concept of neuroplasticity was met with skepticism. For much of the 20th century, scientists believed that the adult brain was fixed and unchangeable. This view began to change with the pioneering work of Santiago Ramón y Cajal, who first suggested that the brain could reorganize itself. However, it wasn't until the late 20th century that the term "neuroplasticity" was coined, and the concept gained widespread acceptance. Early studies, such as those by neuroscientist Michael Merzenich, demonstrated that the brain could change its structure in response to learning and experience. These discoveries revolutionized our understanding of the brain and opened up new possibilities for treating neurological conditions.

The evolution of neuroplasticity from a controversial idea to a well-established scientific theory has profound implications for practical applications. Today, we know that neuroplasticity plays a crucial role in rehabilitation after brain injuries, such as strokes, and in managing neurological conditions like depression and anxiety. It also underscores the importance of lifelong learning and mental stimulation in maintaining cognitive health as we age.

Neuroplasticity is the brain's remarkable ability to adapt and change. It is at the heart of our ability to grow and evolve, from learning a new language to recovering from a stroke or simply adapting to new experiences; understanding and leveraging this incredible capability can unlock new potential and improve your quality of life.

1.2 THE SCIENCE BEHIND NEUROPLASTICITY: HOW THE BRAIN REWIRES ITSELF

Neural pathways and connections are the fundamental elements of neuroplasticity. You can think of neural pathways as the brain's version of muscle memory. When you repeat an action or thought, the neural pathways associated with that activity become stronger and more efficient. For instance, when you practice the piano, your brain strengthens the connections between neurons related to finger movement, auditory processing, and muscle coordination. Over time, this repetition makes playing the piano almost second nature. Conversely, if you stop practicing, those neural pathways can weaken—a phenomenon known as the "use it or lose it" phenomenon mentioned earlier. This principle is akin to an athlete who, after taking an extended break from training, finds their muscles not as strong as they once were. The same happens in the brain, highlighting the importance of consistent mental engagement.

Your brain undergoes structural changes when you engage in new activities or learn new information. For this reason, experiences and learning are potent drivers of neuroplasticity. Let's take another example of juggling. Studies have shown that learning to juggle increases the gray matter in areas of the brain involved in visual and motor coordination. Similarly, meditation has been found to thicken the cortical regions related to attention and sensory processing. In both scenarios, these changes underscore how varied experiences and continual learning can reshape the brain. For instance, someone learning a new language will develop new neural connections that enhance their ability to understand and produce speech in that language. This adaptability is crucial for acquiring new skills and improving cognitive functions.

Neuroplasticity also plays a critical role in recovery from brain injuries. When a specific brain area is damaged, other parts of the brain can often compensate by reorganizing and taking over the lost functions. For example, individuals who have suffered strokes usually undergo rehabilitation that involves repetitive exercises. These exercises are designed to help the brain rewire itself, allowing undamaged areas to assume the functions of the damaged regions. This remarkable ability of the brain to adapt and reorganize is a testament to its resilience and plasticity. Consider a person relearning to walk after a stroke. Their brain forms new pathways to control movement through repetitive physical therapy, gradually restoring their mobility.

Critical periods in neuroplasticity refer to specific times in life when the brain is particularly receptive to environmental stimuli. These periods are most prominent in early childhood, when the brain is highly adaptable and capable of forming new connections rapidly. For example, children learn languages much more quickly than adults because their brains are in a critical period for language acquisition. However, neuroplasticity is not confined to these periods. It continues throughout life, albeit at a slower pace. Through continuous learning and mental stimulation, adults can still enhance their brain's plasticity. An inspiring example is older adults learning to play a musical instrument or taking up a new hobby, demonstrating that the brain retains its ability to change and grow even in later years.

Reflection Exercise: Identify Your Neural Pathways

Take a moment to think about a skill you've mastered, like driving a car or cooking a favorite recipe. Reflect on how your brain has strengthened the neural pathways associated with that skill through repetition. Consider areas where you can form new neural pathways. Write down a new skill or habit you want to develop and outline a plan for consistent practice. This exercise will help you understand the "use it or lose it" principle, reinforcing the importance of regular mental engagement.

In essence, the science behind neuroplasticity reveals a dynamic, adaptable brain capable of significant change. Whether through repetition, new experiences, recovery from injury, or taking advantage of critical periods, our brains are continually rewiring themselves. This adaptability allows us to learn new skills, recover from setbacks, and improve our cognitive functions. Understanding these mechanisms empowers us to actively engage in practices that enhance our brain's plasticity, leading to a richer, more fulfilling life.

1.3 DEBUNKING MYTHS: WHAT NEUROPLASTICITY IS AND ISN'T

One of the most pervasive myths about neuroplasticity is that it only occurs in children. While it's true that young brains are incredibly malleable, the idea that adults can't benefit from neuroplastic changes is simply false. The brain's ability to reorganize itself is a lifelong process. Adults can form new neural connections, learn new skills, and adapt to new environments if they choose to. For instance, consider an adult who decides to learn a new language or take up a musical instrument later in life. Their brain undergoes structural changes to accommodate these new skills, just as they would in a child. The difference lies in the speed and efficiency of these changes, which may be slower in adults, but the potential for growth remains robust.

Another common misconception is that neuroplasticity can cure all forms of brain damage. While neuroplasticity offers incredible potential for recovery and adaptation, it has limits. For example, severe brain injuries may result in permanent deficits that neuroplasticity alone cannot fully remedy. However, it can significantly aid recovery by helping the brain compensate for lost functions. Take the case mentioned earlier of stroke rehabilitation: targeted exercises can help the brain rewire to regain motor skills, but this process is often slow and requires sustained effort. While neuroplasticity can facilitate remarkable improvements, it is not a panacea for all neurological conditions.

Popular media and self-help books often oversimplify or exaggerate the concept of neuroplasticity. You might have heard headlines claiming you can "rewire your brain in just 30 days" or "completely transform your mind with simple tricks." These claims are regularly misleading. Neuroplasticity is a complex, gradual process requiring consistent effort and the right conditions, where quick fixes and miraculous transformations are unrealistic. For example, while engaging in brain-training games can be beneficial, they are not a substitute for comprehensive cognitive activities that involve physical exercise, social interactions, and continuous learning. Oversimplifying neuroplasticity sets unrealistic expectations and undermines the genuine potential it holds for meaningful change.

The scientific consensus on neuroplasticity is both encouraging and realistic. Researchers agree that the brain's ability to change and adapt is a powerful tool for cognitive enhancement and recovery from injury. Studies show that physical exercise, mindfulness meditation, and continuous learning can promote neuroplastic changes. For instance, a study published in *Nature* demonstrated that even short-term mindfulness meditation could lead to structural changes in the brain areas associated with attention and emotional regulation. However, researchers also acknowledge the limitations of the brain's plasticity, which is influenced by factors such as age, genetics, and the severity of any damage. While neuroplasticity can lead to significant improvements, it is not a cure-all and requires a balanced, evidence-based approach to achieve the best results.

Neuroplasticity is a remarkable phenomenon, but it's crucial to approach it with a balanced perspective. By understanding its capabilities and limitations, we can better appreciate how to incorporate its principles into our lives. Whether it's debunking myths, recognizing the limits, or critiquing oversimplifications, a clear, realistic view of neuroplasticity allows us to harness its potential effectively.

This awareness empowers us to make informed decisions about our cognitive health, ensuring that we engage in practices that genuinely enhance our brain's flexibility and resilience.

1.4 THE ROLE OF NEUROTRANSMITTERS IN NEUROPLASTICITY

Understanding neurotransmitters is crucial when discussing neuroplasticity. Neurotransmitters are chemical messengers in the brain that transmit signals from one neuron to another across synapses. Imagine them as the brain's postal service, delivering messages instructing various parts of the brain and body on how to function. There are many types of neurotransmitters, each with a specific role. For instance, dopamine is involved in reward and motivation, serotonin affects mood and social behavior, and BDNF (brain-derived neurotrophic factor) supports existing neurons' survival and encourages new ones' growth. These neurotransmitters facilitate the brain's reorganization ability, making them key players in neuroplasticity.

Neurotransmitters like dopamine, serotonin, and BDNF uniquely promote neuroplastic changes. Dopamine, often referred to as the "feel-good" neurotransmitter, is vital for learning and motivation. When you achieve something rewarding, your brain releases dopamine, strengthening the neural pathways associated with that action. This is why positive reinforcement is so effective in learning new skills. Serotonin, on the other hand, helps regulate mood and emotion. Higher serotonin levels can enhance mood and cognitive functions, creating a more conducive environment for neuroplastic changes. BDNF is particularly significant because it promotes the growth of new neurons and synapses, supporting the brain's ability to adapt and learn. Think of BDNF as a fertilizer for the brain, encouraging its growth and strengthening neural connections.

External factors like diet, exercise, and stress significantly impact neurotransmitter levels and neuroplasticity. A balanced diet rich in omega-3 fatty acids, antioxidants, and other essential nutrients can boost neurotransmitter production and support brain health. Foods like salmon, blueberries, and walnuts enhance cognitive functions by promoting neurotransmitter activity. Regular exercise is another potent modulator of neurotransmitters. Physical activity increases the production of BDNF, dopamine, and serotonin, thereby enhancing mood, motivation, and cognitive functions. Chronic stress, however, can have the opposite effect, depleting neurotransmitter levels, impairing cognitive functions, and reducing the brain's plasticity. Managing stress through mindfulness, yoga, or other relaxation techniques can help maintain healthy neurotransmitter levels, promoting a resilient and adaptable brain.

Recent research provides compelling evidence of the link between neurotransmitter activity and changes in brain plasticity. A study published in the journal *Nature Neuroscience* found that regular aerobic exercise significantly increased BDNF levels in participants, leading to improved memory and cognitive functions. The study involved a group of middle-aged adults participating in a six-month aerobic exercise program. Compared to a control group that did not exercise, the participants showed notable improvements in memory and cognitive flexibility, highlighting the role of BDNF in facilitating these changes. Another study focused on the effects of mindfulness meditation on neurotransmitter levels. Participants who engaged in an eight-week mindfulness meditation program showed increased serotonin levels and improved mood regulation linked to structural changes in brain regions associated with emotional processing and attention.

Case Study: The Impact of Exercise on Neurotransmitters

Think of a group of sedentary adults who began a regular exercise routine. Over six months, they engaged in moderate aerobic activities like walking and cycling. Researchers measured their BDNF, dopamine, and serotonin levels before and after the program. The results were striking. Participants showed a significant increase in BDNF levels, correlating with enhanced memory and learning capabilities. Dopamine levels also rose, leading to better motivation and mood. Serotonin levels improved, reducing symptoms of anxiety and depression. This case study underscores the profound impact of physical activity on neurotransmitter levels and, by extension, neuroplasticity, highlighting the importance of integrating regular exercise into your routine to support brain health and cognitive functions.

Understanding the role of neurotransmitters in neuroplasticity reveals how interconnected our brain's chemical environment is with our ability to learn, adapt, and grow. Maintaining a healthy diet, exercising regularly, and managing stress can influence neurotransmitter levels and enhance your brain's plasticity. These insights deepen our understanding of neuroplasticity and provide practical strategies for improving cognitive health and overall well-being.

1.5 SYNAPTIC PLASTICITY: THE KEY MECHANISMS OF LEARNING AND MEMORY

Synaptic plasticity lies at the heart of how our brains learn and remember. Synapses are the communication points between neurons, similar to intersections where traffic signals control the flow of information. By strengthening these synapses through repeated use, we make it easier for information to travel along these pathways. Conversely, when we don't use them, they weaken. This process is akin to how a well-trodden path in a forest becomes easier to navigate over time while an unused trail becomes overgrown and harder to traverse. Synaptic plasticity, therefore, is the brain's ability to strengthen or weaken these synaptic connections based on activity levels.

The biological mechanisms behind synaptic plasticity can be boiled down to two key processes: Long-term potentiation (LTP) and long-term depression (LTD). LTP is the process by which synapses become stronger with frequent activation. Like lifting weights at the gym, the more you lift, the stronger your muscles become. Similarly, the more frequently a synapse is activated, the stronger the connection becomes.

On the other hand, LTD is the process by which synapses weaken when they are rarely used. Think of it as the brain's way of pruning away unused connections, much like how a gardener trims away dead branches to promote the growth of healthy ones. These processes ensure that our brains remain efficient, reinforcing beneficial connections while eliminating those that are no longer needed.

Synaptic plasticity is directly tied to our ability to learn and remember. When you memorize a piece of information or learn a new skill, your brain undergoes synaptic changes to store this new knowledge. For example, when you learn to play a new song on the guitar, the synapses involved in finger movement, auditory processing, and muscle coordination are strengthened. This makes it easier to play the song the next time, as the neural pathways are more robust. Similarly, when you memorize a fact for an exam, the synapses associated with that piece of information are strengthened, making it easier to recall during the test. This continuous process of strengthening and weakening synapses allows us to learn new things and retain information over time.

Recent research has shed light on innovative ways to enhance learning and memory through targeted synaptic modification. One study published in the journal *Cell Reports* found that specific types of brain stimulation could enhance LTP, leading to improved memory retention. Participants who underwent targeted brain stimulation showed a significantly enhanced ability to recall information compared to the control group. This finding suggests that non-invasive brain stimulation techniques could be used to boost synaptic plasticity and improve cognitive functions. Another study focused on the role of sleep in synaptic plasticity. Researchers discovered that deep sleep is crucial in consolidating memories and strengthening synaptic connections. Participants who had a good night's sleep after learning a new task showed better performance and retention than those who did not, highlighting the importance of sleep in optimizing synaptic plasticity and cognitive performance.

Practical Application: Enhancing Synaptic Plasticity Through Daily Activities

Try incorporating activities into your daily routine that promote synaptic plasticity. Engage in challenging tasks stimulating synaptic changes and enhancing cognitive functions, such as learning a new language, playing a musical instrument, or solving puzzles. Additionally, ensure you get adequate sleep to consolidate memories and strengthen synaptic connections. Regular physical exercise can also boost synaptic plasticity by increasing the production of BDNF. This protein supports the growth and differentiation of new neurons and synapses. Integrating these practices into your daily life can enhance your brain's ability to learn and remember.

Understanding synaptic plasticity provides valuable insights into how our brains function and adapt. By recognizing the processes of LTP and LTD, we can appreciate the dynamic nature of our neural connections. This knowledge empowers us to take proactive steps to enhance our cognitive abilities, ensuring that our brains remain flexible and capable of learning throughout our lives.

1.6 NEUROGENESIS: UNDERSTANDING BRAIN GROWTH ACROSS LIFESPAN

Neurogenesis is the process by which new neurons are generated in the brain. This phenomenon continues throughout adulthood, contrary to the long-held belief that we are born with a fixed number of neurons. This process plays a crucial role in neuroplasticity, contributing to the brain's ability to adapt, learn, and recover. New neurons are primarily generated in the hippocampus, a region associated with memory and spatial navigation. Think of neurogenesis as the brain's way of keeping itself fresh and resilient, much like how a garden thrives with the continuous planting of new seeds. The benefits of neurogenesis are manifold, including enhanced memory, improved mood, and greater cognitive flexibility, which are vital for maintaining brain health as we age.

The hippocampus is the most well-known site of neurogenesis in the adult brain. This seahorse-shaped structure is deeply involved in forming and retrieving memories and navigating through space. When new neurons are generated in the hippocampus, they integrate into existing neural circuits, enhancing the brain's capacity to form new memories and improve spatial navigation. Studies have shown that activities like learning a new route or engaging in complex puzzles can stimulate neurogenesis in the hippocampus. This continuous generation of new neurons ensures that the hippocampus remains functional and capable of adapting to new information and experiences, much like how updating software keeps a computer running efficiently.

Several factors influence neurogenesis, either promoting or inhibiting the process. Age is a significant factor; as we age, the rate of neurogenesis naturally declines. However, this does not mean that neurogenesis stops altogether. Physical exercise is one of the most potent promoters of neurogenesis. Aerobic activities like running and swimming have been shown to increase the production of BDNF, a protein supporting new neuron growth. Diet also plays a crucial role. Foods rich in omega-3 fatty acids, antioxidants, and flavonoids, such as fatty fish, berries, and dark chocolate, can enhance neurogenesis.

On the other hand, chronic stress and a poor diet can inhibit the process. Stress hormones like cortisol can damage the hippocampus and reduce the production of new neurons. Therefore, managing stress through mindfulness, getting adequate sleep, and maintaining a balanced diet is vital for promoting neurogenesis.

The implications of neurogenesis for aging and cognitive health are profound. Active neurogenesis is linked to reduced rates of cognitive decline in older adults. A study published in the journal *Nature Medicine* found that older adults who engaged in regular physical exercise showed higher levels of neurogenesis and better cognitive performance than their sedentary peers. These findings suggest that lifestyle choices can significantly impact the brain's ability to generate new neurons, influencing cognitive health. By maintaining a lifestyle that promotes neurogenesis and adopting habits that support brain health, like regular exercise and effective stress management, older adults can potentially stave off conditions like Alzheimer's disease and other forms of dementia.

Neurogenesis is not merely a fascinating scientific concept; it has real-world implications for how we live our lives. By understanding the factors that influence the generation of new neurons, we can take proactive steps to enhance our brain's plasticity and overall health. Whether it's through physical exercise, a balanced diet, or stress management, our daily choices can significantly impact our brain's ability to grow and adapt. This understanding and associated actions empower us to take control of our cognitive health, ensuring that our brains remain resilient and capable of learning throughout our lives.

1.7 TEST YOUR KNOWLEDGE

To help solidify your understanding and ensure that you are ready to apply neuroplasticity principles in your daily life, this section features a quiz designed to reinforce critical concepts and practical applications. This will test your knowledge and provide an interactive way to engage with the material, helping you internalize the lessons from this chapter.

Question 1: True or False: Neuroplasticity only occurs during childhood, and the adult brain cannot change.

Question 2: Multiple Choice: Which neurotransmitter is often called the "feel-good" chemical and is crucial for learning and motivation?

A) Serotonin
B) Dopamine
C) BDNF
D) Acetylcholine

Question 3: True or False: Chronic stress can inhibit neurogenesis and negatively affect brain plasticity.

Question 4: Multiple Choice: Which area of the brain primarily generates new neurons in adults?

A) Cerebellum
B) Hippocampus
C) Amygdala
D) Prefrontal Cortex

Question 5: True or False: Synaptic plasticity refers to the brain's ability to strengthen or weaken synapses, the communication points between neurons.

Question 6: Multiple Choice: Which activity has been shown to increase the production of brain-derived neurotrophic factor (BDNF)?

A) Watching TV
B) Aerobic exercise
C) Eating junk food
D) Sitting still

Question 7: True or False: The concept of neuroplasticity was universally accepted as soon as it was introduced.

Question 8: Multiple Choice: What is the critical role of deep sleep in neuroplasticity?

A) It weakens neural connections
B) It consolidates memories and strengthens synaptic connections

C) It eliminates all learned information

D) It has no impact on neuroplasticity

Question 9: True or False: Learning new skills can lead to structural changes in the brain, enhancing cognitive functions.

Question 10: Multiple Choice: Which factor does NOT promote neurogenesis?

A) Physical exercise

B) Chronic stress

C) A balanced diet

D) Learning new skills

Answers:

1. False
2. B) Dopamine
3. True
4. B) Hippocampus
5. True
6. B) Aerobic exercise
7. False
8. B) It consolidates memories and strengthens synaptic connections
9. True
10. B) Chronic stress

Reflecting on what you've learned so far, think about how these concepts can be applied to your own life. Analyze the activities you engage in daily and how they might be influencing your brain's plasticity. Are there small changes you can make to promote better brain health? It could be incorporating a new exercise routine, practicing mindfulness, or making different dietary choices. Whatever your preference, these small steps can have a significant impact over time.

Understanding neuroplasticity isn't just about grasping scientific concepts; it's about recognizing the incredible potential for growth and change within each of us. The brain's ability to adapt and reorganize itself offers a powerful tool for enhancing cognitive functions, recovering from injuries, and improving overall mental health. Each principle you've encountered in this chapter contributes to a broader understanding of how to nurture and enhance your brain's plasticity.

As you move forward, remember that the brain's capacity for change is lifelong. Whether learning a new language, picking up a musical instrument, or simply engaging in regular physical activity, each action contributes to the ongoing reshaping of your neural landscape. Embrace these growth opportunities, and you'll find that the benefits extend far beyond mere knowledge—they can transform your way of living.

Now that you have a solid foundation, you're well-prepared to explore more detailed aspects of neuroplasticity and how to apply them practically in your daily life. The journey to optimizing brain health and cognitive function is ongoing, and it starts with the principles you've learned here. The power to change and grow lies within your brain, waiting to be unlocked, so let's continue our journey.

CHAPTER TWO

NEUROPLASTICITY AND LIFESTYLE

I magine waking up each morning feeling sharper, more focused, and ready to tackle the day's challenges with clarity and vigor. This isn't a far-fetched dream but a reality for those who understand and implement the principles of neuroplasticity in their daily lives. A pivotal aspect of this transformation lies in our lifestyle choices, mainly what we eat. Food is more than just fuel; it's the building block of our brain's health and ability to rewire itself. The connection between nutrition and neuroplasticity is profound, and by making conscious dietary choices, you can significantly enhance your brain's ability to adapt, learn, and thrive.

2.1 NUTRITION AND SUPPLEMENTS THAT BOOST BRAIN HEALTH

Nutrition plays a crucial role in brain health and neuroplasticity. The foods you consume provide the essential nutrients that support neural growth and synaptic plasticity. For instance, omega-3 fatty acids found in fish like salmon and mackerel are vital for maintaining the structural integrity of your brain cells. These fatty acids help build cell membranes in the brain and have anti-inflammatory properties that protect brain cells from damage. Antioxidants, abundant in berries, nuts, and dark chocolate, combat oxidative stress that can impair cognitive functions. Proteins in lean meats, eggs, and legumes provide amino acids essential for neurotransmitter production. These nutrients collectively contribute to a robust neural network, enhancing your brain's ability to form new connections and stay resilient against cognitive decline.

The impact of specific diets on brain plasticity is well-documented. The Mediterranean diet, rich in vegetables, fruits, whole grains, olive oil, beans, and fish, has been associated with fewer signs of Alzheimer's disease and other forms of cognitive decline. A study involving 581 participants revealed that higher adherence to the Mediterranean diet correlated with fewer amyloid plaques associated with Alzheimer's disease. The Mediterranean-DASH intervention for Neurodegenerative Delay (MIND) diet, which emphasizes green leafy vegetables, berries, beans, nuts, and weekly servings of fish, has shown similar benefits. Both diets include olive oil, whole grains, and small amounts of wine while limiting red meat. These diets are proven to support overall health and provide the nutrients necessary for maintaining and enhancing neuroplasticity.

Nutrient-rich diets, such as those with omega-3 fatty acids, antioxidants, and proteins, are essential for neural growth and plasticity. Omega-3 fatty acids, particularly docosahexaenoic acid (DHA), are crucial for brain development and function. Foods rich in omega-3s include fatty fish, flaxseeds, chia seeds, and walnuts. Antioxidants in vibrant fruits and vegetables like blueberries, spinach, and kale protect the brain from oxidative stress and inflammation. Proteins, broken down into amino acids during digestion, are necessary for neurotransmitter synthesis. Lean meats, eggs, dairy products, and plant-based sources like beans and lentils provide the amino acids required for optimal brain function.

Supplements can also support brain health and neuroplasticity. When selecting supplements, looking for those with proven efficacy is essential. Nootropics, often referred to as "smart drugs," are compounds that enhance cognitive function. Common nootropics include caffeine, L-theanine, and creatine, which have been shown to improve focus, memory, and mental clarity. Adaptogens, such as ashwagandha, Rhodiola, and ginseng, help the body adapt to stress and support overall brain health. These supplements can enhance neuroplasticity by promoting a balanced and resilient neural environment. For instance, L-theanine, found in green tea, has been shown to improve attention and reaction time. At the same time, ashwagandha can reduce stress and anxiety, creating a more conducive environment for neuroplastic changes.

Please always consult a health provider before using any supplements, especially if you have health conditions or are on medication. The use of supplements is at your own risk.

However, foods like excessive sugars and processed fats are not beneficial for brain health and can negatively impact neuroplasticity. High sugar intake can lead to insulin resistance, which has been linked to cognitive decline and an increased risk of Alzheimer's disease. Processed fats, such as trans fats, can cause inflammation and oxidative stress, damaging brain cells and impairing cognitive functions. Overly processed foods, often high in unhealthy fats and sugars, can lead to obesity, diabetes, and cardiovascular diseases, which are risk factors for cognitive decline. Avoiding these harmful foods and focusing on a diet rich in whole, nutrient-dense foods can significantly enhance your brain's health and ability to adapt and grow.

Incorporating brain-boosting foods into your daily meals doesn't have to be complicated; you can start by including various colorful fruits and vegetables in your diet. Aim for at least five servings of vegetables and two servings of fruit daily. Add fatty fish to your meals a few times a week and incorporate nuts and seeds as snacks. Consider trying the Mediterranean or MIND diet for its well-documented benefits on brain health. For a simple, brain-boosting breakfast, try a smoothie made with spinach, blueberries, a tablespoon of flaxseed, and a scoop of protein powder. A salad with mixed greens, grilled salmon, avocado, and a drizzle of olive oil can be delicious and nutritious for lunch. Dinner could include a quinoa bowl with roasted vegetables, chickpeas, and a sprinkle of nuts. These small dietary changes can significantly impact your brain's flexibility and resilience.

By understanding the profound connection between nutrition and neuroplasticity, you can make informed choices that support your brain's health and cognitive functions. With the right foods and supplements, you can enhance your brain's ability to adapt, learn, and thrive, ensuring a vibrant and fulfilling life.

2.2 THE IMPACT OF PHYSICAL EXERCISE ON BRAIN PLASTICITY

Regular physical exercise isn't just about staying fit or losing weight; it's also a powerful way to boost your brain's health and enhance neuroplasticity. When you exercise, your body produces a BDNF protein, which acts like a fertilizer for your brain. It promotes the growth of new neurons and strengthens existing connections, making your brain more adaptable and resilient. As mentioned in the previous chapter, your body produces BDNF primarily in the hippocampus, an area crucial for learning and memory. The more you engage in physical activities, the more BDNF is released, facilitating better cognitive function and mental flexibility.

Research has shown that regular physical exercise can lead to significant neuroplastic changes. A study published in the journal *Nature Neuroscience* found that participants who engaged in aerobic exercises, such as running or cycling, exhibited increased levels of BDNF and improved memory performance. Another study on older adults revealed that those who participated in a six-month aerobic exercise program showed enhanced cognitive functions and increased hippocampal volume, illustrating the profound impact of exercise on brain health. These findings underscore the importance of incorporating physical activity into your daily routine to promote brain plasticity and cognitive wellness.

Different types of exercise offer various benefits for neuroplasticity. Aerobic exercises like running, swimming, and cycling are practical in boosting BDNF levels and enhancing overall cognitive function. Resistance or strength training, such as lifting weights or using resistance bands, also has significant benefits. It helps retain muscle mass and strength as you age and improves brain health, mood regulation, and stress resilience. Yoga and tai chi combine physical movement with mindfulness, promoting relaxation and mental clarity while reducing neuroinflammation. These activities and others encourage the brain to form new connections, enhancing physical and psychological health.

To maximize the neuroplastic benefits of exercise, it's essential to integrate a variety of physical activities into your daily routine. Here is an example routine: Start with moderate aerobic exercises, such as brisk walking or cycling, for at least 30 minutes a day, five days a week. If you're new to exercise, begin with short, manageable sessions and gradually increase the duration and intensity. Incorporate resistance training twice a week, focusing on major muscle groups. Simple exercises like bodyweight squats, push-ups, and resistance band exercises can be effective. Additionally, flexibility and balance exercises like yoga or tai chi should be included to promote overall well-being. A combination of these practices enhances physical fitness and supports cognitive health and neuroplasticity.

To make the learnings from this chapter more personalized for you, try setting up a weekly exercise schedule to ensure consistency. For example, you might go for a brisk walk on Mondays, Wednesdays, and Fridays and engage in strength training on Tuesdays and Thursdays. Try a yoga or tai chi session on weekends to relax and rejuvenate. The key is to find activities you enjoy, making it easier to stick to your routine. Consistency is crucial for reaping the neuroplastic benefits of exercise, so it's important to make physical activity a regular part of your life.

2.3 SLEEP AND NEUROPLASTICITY: HOW REST REWIRES THE BRAIN

Sleep is not merely a passive state of rest; it is a dynamic period of brain activity that significantly contributes to neuroplasticity. One of the critical mechanisms by which sleep affects neuroplasticity is memory consolidation and synaptic pruning. Memory consolidation is the process of transforming short-term memories into long-term ones. During sleep, especially deep sleep and REM sleep, the brain replays the day's experiences, strengthening the synaptic connections that are most relevant while weakening those that are less important. This process ensures that valuable information is retained while extraneous details are discarded, making room for new learning. On the other hand, synaptic pruning is like a gardener trimming away dead branches to allow healthy ones to flourish. The brain optimizes its neural network by removing weaker synaptic connections, enhancing overall cognitive efficiency.

Recent research illuminates the critical role of sleep in maintaining and enhancing brain plasticity. A study published in Nature Neuroscience journal demonstrated that sleep stabilizes and strengthens memories rather than merely protecting them from interference. Participants who slept after learning new information showed significantly better recall than those who stayed awake, defending the role of sleep in memory consolidation. Another study found that sleep promotes the growth of dendritic spines, small protrusions on neurons that facilitate synaptic connections. Both findings underscore the importance of sleep in reinforcing neural pathways and fostering a resilient, adaptable brain.

The negative impact of sleep deprivation on brain function and plasticity is significant. Chronic lack of sleep impairs cognitive functions such as learning, memory, and decision-making. When you are sleep-deprived, your brain's ability to consolidate memories and prune synapses is significantly compromised. This leads to a buildup of irrelevant information and a weakening of essential neural connections, resulting in cognitive fog and decreased mental agility. Moreover, sleep deprivation increases the production of stress hormones like cortisol, which can damage the hippocampus, a region critical for memory and learning. Over time, chronic sleep deprivation can lead to more severe cognitive decline and an increased risk of neurodegenerative diseases.

Optimizing sleep for brain health involves adopting habits and using tools that promote high-quality rest. Establishing a regular sleep schedule by going to bed and waking up at the same time each day helps regulate your body's internal clock. Creating a sleep-conducive environment is crucial; ensure your bedroom is cool, dark, and quiet. Limiting exposure to screens before bedtime can help, as the blue light emitted by phones and computers can inter-fere with the production of melatonin, a hormone that regulates sleep. Relaxing activities such as reading, taking a warm bath, or practicing mindfulness meditation can prepare your mind and body for sleep.

Additional sleep optimizing variables may include supplements like melatonin and magnesium, which can support sleep quality, but it's essential to use them wisely and consult a healthcare provider. Melatonin can help regulate sleep-wake cycles, especially if you have trouble falling asleep. Magnesium, known for its muscle-relaxing properties, can promote a sense of calm and ease anxiety, making it easier to drift off. Tools like white noise machines can mask disruptive sounds, and weighted blankets can provide a comforting sense of security that promotes deeper sleep.

For those struggling with specific sleep issues, consider trying tech-niques like cognitive-behavioral therapy for insomnia, which addresses the thoughts and behaviors that disrupt sleep. Keeping a sleep journal can help you track patterns and identify factors contributing to poor sleep. This journal could include notes on bedtime routines, diet, exercise, and stress levels, providing valu-able insights into what works best for you. Integrating these practices and tools into your routine can enhance your sleep quality, supporting your brain's ability to adapt and promoting plasticity.

2.4 STRESS MANAGEMENT AND ITS EFFECTS ON BRAIN WIRING

Chronic stress is a persistent state over an extended period, often triggered by factors such as work pressure, financial worries, or personal relationships. This type of stress can wreak havoc on your brain, particularly affecting the hippocampus and prefrontal cortex. The hippocampus, responsible for memory and learning, shrinks under prolonged stress, impairing its ability to function effectively. The prefrontal cortex, which governs decision-making, emotional regulation, and executive function, suffers as well. Chronic stress disrupts the balance of neurotransmitters, leading to cognitive decline and emotional instability. Imagine your brain as a finely tuned orchestra; chronic stress is like a disruptive noise that throws the entire symphony out of harmony, making it difficult for the brain to function optimally.

Managing stress effectively can significantly enhance neuroplasticity, allowing your brain to maintain adaptability and resilience. Mindfulness is one powerful technique that involves paying attention to the present moment without judgment. Focusing on your breath or bodily sensations can calm the mind and reduce stress, fostering a conducive environment for neuroplastic changes. Gratitude journaling is another effective method. By regularly writing down things you're grateful for, you shift your focus from stressors to positive aspects of your life, which can improve your mood and cognitive flexibility. Meditation, a practice of sustained focus and relaxation, has been shown to increase grey matter density in the brain, particularly in areas associated with attention and emotional regulation. Deep breathing exercises like diaphragmatic breathing can activate the parasympathetic nervous system, reducing stress hormones and promoting relaxation. Progressive muscle relaxation involves tensing and slowly relaxing different muscle groups, which can help alleviate physical tension and calm the mind.

Balancing stress involves reducing it and managing it to foster resilience. Think of stress as a double-edged sword. While chronic stress is harmful, short bursts of stress, known as acute stress, can enhance neuroplasticity by preparing the brain to adapt to new challenges. The key is to find a balance and establish a routine with stress-reducing activities, which can help you manage chronic stress and leverage acute stress for growth. For instance, integrating mindfulness practices into your daily routine, setting aside time for hobbies, and ensuring regular physical activity can create a balanced approach to stress. This balance helps maintain cognitive flexibility and resilience, allowing your brain to adapt and thrive in various situations.

Reflection Section: Personal Stress Management Plan

Take a moment to reflect on your current stress levels. Identify your life's primary sources of stress and consider how they might impact your cognitive functions and overall well-being. Write down three stress management techniques you can incorporate into your daily routine. These could include mindfulness practices, gratitude journaling, or regular physical exercise. Set specific, achievable goals for each technique, like practicing mindfulness for ten minutes each morning or writing in a gratitude journal before bed. By creating a personalized stress management plan that works best for your schedule, you can take proactive steps to enhance your brain health and neuroplasticity.

Case examples help to provide compelling evidence of the impact of effective stress management on brain plasticity. Consider the story of Sarah, a high school teacher who experienced severe burnout from the demands of her job. She began practicing mindfulness meditation and gratitude journaling daily. Over several months, Sarah noticed significant improvements in her mood, focus, and memory. A study published in *Psychiatry Research* supports similar outcomes, showing that participants who engaged in an eight-week mindfulness program exhibited increased grey matter density in the hippocampus and prefrontal cortex. Another case involves John, a corporate executive who used progressive muscle relaxation and deep breathing exercises to manage his work-related stress. These practices reduced his stress levels and enhanced his decision-making and problem-solving abilities, highlighting the practical benefits of stress management techniques.

By understanding the profound impact of stress on brain wiring and implementing effective stress management techniques, you can also foster an environment that supports neuroplasticity and cognitive health. This proactive approach helps maintain the brain's adaptability and resilience, ensuring it remains capable of learning and thriving throughout your life.

2.5 THE BRAIN-ENHANCING BENEFITS OF REGULAR MEDITATION

Meditation has long been touted for its profound effects on the mind, and recent scientific findings have solidified its role in enhancing brain structure. Regular meditation practices, such as mindfulness, have increased grey matter density in areas of the brain associated with attention, emotion regulation, and mental flexibility. You can think of these areas as the brain's focus and emotional resilience control centers. When you meditate regularly, you essentially exercise these control centers, making them stronger and more efficient. This increased grey matter density helps you stay focused and calm in stressful situations and enhances your overall cognitive function and wellness. Meditation also fosters mindfulness, a state of being fully present and engaged in the moment, which has been linked to improved mental health and life satisfaction.

Scientific studies have provided robust evidence supporting the cognitive benefits of meditation. For example, a study from *Harvard Medical School* revealed that regular meditation could reduce the size of the amygdala, the brain's fear center, which helps in reducing stress and anxiety levels. These findings reinforce the validity of meditation as a powerful tool for enhancing neuroplasticity and overall brain health. They show that meditation is not just a mental exercise but a physical one that brings about measurable changes in the brain's structure.

Exploring different meditation practices can provide various benefits for neuroplasticity. Some practical techniques include mindfulness meditation, which involves paying attention to your breath, thoughts, and sensations without judgment. This practice helps to improve focus and emotional regulation. Transcendental meditation, which uses a mantra or repeated words, can create deep relaxation and reduce stress. Loving-kindness meditation involves directing feelings of love and compassion towards yourself and others, which can enhance emotional resilience and empathy. Focused attention meditation, where you concentrate on a single object or thought, can improve your ability to maintain attention and reduce mind-wandering. Each of these practices impacts different brain areas, promoting overall cognitive health.

Starting a meditation practice can seem daunting, but it doesn't have to be. You can begin by setting aside just five to ten minutes each day for meditation. Find a quiet space where you won't be disturbed. Sit comfortably with your back straight and your hands resting on your lap. Close your eyes and take a few deep breaths to center yourself. You can start with mindfulness meditation by focusing on your breath. Notice the sensation of the air entering and leaving your nostrils. If your mind wanders, gently bring your focus back to your breath without judgment. Over time, you can gradually increase the duration of your meditation sessions. After a few weeks, you may notice improvements in your ability to focus, manage stress, and regulate your emotions.

To help you get started, here's a beginner-friendly meditation schedule. Aim for five minutes of mindfulness meditation each day for the first week. In the second week, increase to ten minutes. By the third week, you can experiment with different types of meditation, such as loving-kindness or focused attention, for ten minutes each day. Keep a meditation journal to track your progress and note any mood, focus, or stress changes. Numerous resources are available to support your practice, including meditation apps like Headspace and Calm, which offer guided meditations and mindfulness exercises tailored to various needs and experience levels. These tools can provide you with additional structure and support, making establishing a consistent meditation routine easier.

2.6 COGNITIVE FLEXIBILITY THROUGH HOBBIES AND CREATIVE PURSUITS

Engaging in hobbies and creative pursuits like painting, music, and writing can significantly enhance your brain's health by challenging it in new and complex ways. When you pick up a paintbrush or strum a guitar, your brain activates multiple regions simultaneously. This kind of activity is similar to a full-body workout for your brain. Painting, for instance, requires fine motor skills, visual processing, and emotional expression. These activities stimulate neural pathways and promote neuroplasticity, making your brain more adaptable and resilient. Conversely, writing engages language skills, memory recall, and creative thinking, all of which contribute to a more flexible and robust neural network.

There are numerous cognitive benefits to regularly engaging in creative activities, including improving problem-solving skills by encouraging you to think outside the box and find innovative solutions. Enhanced memory is another significant benefit. When you learn a new piece of music or memorize lines for a play, you exercise your memory muscles, making them stronger and more reliable. Greater mental flexibility is also a key advantage. Creative pursuits require you to switch between logical, spatial, or emotional modes of thinking. This constant shifting helps your brain become more agile and adapt to new situations and challenges better.

Research supports the long-term benefits of creative engagement in maintaining cognitive health and promoting neuroplasticity. A study published in the *Journal of Aging and Health* found that older adults who engaged in creative activities like painting and music showed slower cognitive decline than those who did not. Another study in the *Journal of Neuropsychology* revealed that individuals who participated in regular creative writing exercises had better memory retention and cognitive flexibility. These findings under-score the importance of incorporating creative activities into your daily life, showing that engaging in hobbies isn't just a way to pass the time but a crucial element in maintaining and enhancing brain health.

Incorporating more creativity into your life doesn't have to be daunting, even if you don't initially consider yourself "creative." Start with easy, low-barrier entry activities. Try adult coloring books, which allow you to express yourself without the pressure of creating something from scratch. Take up journaling, where you can write about your day and your thoughts or even create fictional stories. Another great option is joining a local community choir or playing a musical instrument. You don't have to be a professional singer or musician to reap the cognitive benefits. The key is finding something you enjoy that challenges your brain in new ways.

To make creativity a regular part of your routine, set aside a specific time dedicated to your chosen activity each day or week. This could be as simple as spending 15 minutes each morning journaling or an hour every weekend painting. If you're pressed for time, look for ways to integrate creativity into your existing routine. For example, listen to a podcast about creative writing during your commute or doodle while on a conference call. The goal is to make creative activities consistent in your life, ensuring your brain is continually challenged and stimulated.

Engaging in creative hobbies enriches your life and significantly enhances your brain's health and neuroplasticity. Challenging your brain in new and complex ways can improve problem-solving skills, enhance memory, and increase mental flexibility. Research supports the long-term cognitive benefits of creative engagement, making it an essential component of a healthy lifestyle. Even if you don't see yourself as creative, there are plenty of low-difficulty activities to help you get started. So, pick up that paintbrush, journal, or instrument and start reaping the cognitive rewards today.

2.7 TEST YOUR KNOWLEDGE

By now, you've explored various lifestyle habits that can significantly enhance your brain's plasticity. From the foods you eat to the exercises you engage in, each element is crucial in ensuring that your brain remains flexible, resilient, and capable of growth. To help solidify your understanding and ensure that you're ready to apply these principles in your daily life, let's test your knowledge with a short quiz. Like before, this will reinforce the critical concepts and provide an interactive way to engage with the material.

Question 1: True or False: Regular meditation can increase grey matter density in areas of the brain associated with attention and emotion regulation.

Question 2: Multiple Choice: Which neurotransmitter is often called the "feel-good" chemical and crucial for learning and motivation?

    A) Serotonin
    B) Dopamine
    C) BDNF
    D) Acetylcholine

Question 3: True or False: Chronic stress can negatively impact neuroplasticity by shrinking the hippocampus and impairing cognitive functions.

Question 4: Multiple Choice: Which exercise is particularly effective in boosting BDNF levels and enhancing overall cognitive function?

A) Yoga
B) Strength training
C) Tai chi
D) Aerobic exercise

Question 5: True or False: Engaging in creative activities like painting and music can improve problem-solving skills and enhance mental flexibility.

Question 6: Multiple Choice: What is the primary role of sleep in neuroplasticity?

A) It weakens neural connections
B) It consolidates memories and prunes synapses
C) It eliminates all learned information
D) It has no impact on neuroplasticity

Question 7: True or False: Mindfulness meditation involves paying attention to your breath, thoughts, and sensations without judgment.

Question 8: Multiple Choice: Which diet is associated with fewer signs of Alzheimer's disease and supports brain plasticity?

A) Keto
B) Mediterranean
C) Carnivore
D) Paleo

Question 9: True or False: Regular physical exercise can lead to significant neuroplastic changes and improve memory performance.

Question 10: Multiple Choice: Which stress management technique involves writing down things you're grateful for?

  A) Deep breathing exercises
  B) Progressive muscle relaxation
  C) Gratitude journaling
  D) Mindfulness meditation

Answers:

1. True
2. B) Dopamine
3. True
4. D) Aerobic exercise
5. True
6. B) It consolidates memories and prunes synapses
7. True
8. B) Mediterranean
9. True
10. C) Gratitude journaling

Reflect on your responses to understand where your strengths lie and which areas may need further exploration. The goal is to test your knowledge and deepen your understanding of how these lifestyle habits contribute to neuroplasticity. To get the full effect of your learnings, try integrating these practices into your daily life, making small, sustainable changes that enhance your brain's health and adaptability.

In the bigger picture, these practices are more than individual habits; they are comprehensive approaches to maintaining and enhancing cognitive functions. As you continue to explore the principles of neuroplasticity, remember that each small step you take contributes to a more resilient and adaptable brain. Embrace the journey of lifelong learning and self-improvement, knowing that every effort you make is a step towards a healthier, more vibrant mind.

Armed with this knowledge, you can explore strategies and interventions to enhance your brain's plasticity further. The next chapter will guide you through practical applications and real-life examples, offering a roadmap to unlock your brain's full potential.

CHAPTER THREE
PRACTICAL APPLICATIONS OF NEUROPLASTICITY

Picture yourself waking up each morning with a clear mind, a sense of purpose, and feeling ready to take on the day. This isn't just wishful thinking; it's the tangible outcome of a well-structured morning routine that leverages the principles of neuroplasticity. Incorporating deliberate practices into your morning can set the tone for the entire day, enhancing cognitive function, focus, and overall mental health. Let's explore how establishing a consistent morning routine can be a game-changer for your brain health.

3.1 MORNING ROUTINES TO BOOST COGNITIVE FUNCTION

Establishing a consistent morning routine is not merely about following a set of rituals; it's about creating a framework that helps you plan your day, enhance discipline, and use your time effectively. When you wake up at the same time each day, you regulate your circadian rhythm, which is your body's internal clock. This consistency aids in aligning your sleep-wake cycles, ensuring you feel more alert and energized throughout the day. Additionally, starting your day with structured activities can help reduce decision fatigue, allowing your brain to focus on more important tasks later on. Small, gradual changes in your morning routine can have a significant impact. You can begin by setting your alarm for the same time each morning and commit to waking up at that time, even on weekends. Over time, this will help your body get accustomed to a regular schedule, making it easier to wake up feeling refreshed.

One of the first steps in a productive morning routine is to wake up early and consistently. Early risers often report higher levels of productivity and mental clarity. When you wake up early, you give yourself a head start on the day, allowing time for activities that prime your brain for optimal performance. Exposure to natural light as soon as possible after waking up can further regulate your circadian rhythm by signaling your brain that it's time to be alert. Try opening your curtains or step outside for a few minutes to soak in the morning sunlight. This simple act can boost your mood and help you feel more awake.

Prioritizing hydration and nutrition upon waking is crucial for optimal brain function. After hours of sleep, your body is naturally dehydrated, and drinking a glass of water first thing in the morning helps rehydrate your system. It is also essential for maintaining cognitive function, as even mild dehydration can impair concentration and short-term memory. Follow this with a balanced breakfast containing proteins, healthy fats, and complex carbohydrates. Avoid sugary foods that can lead to energy crashes later in the day. A nutritious breakfast supports sustained energy levels and provides the necessary nutrients for your brain to function effectively. For instance, you can make scrambled eggs with avocado and whole-grain toast or a smoothie packed with spinach, berries, and a scoop of protein powder for a brain-boosting breakfast.

Incorporating physical and mental exercise into your morning routine can significantly boost cognitive function. Physical activities like walking, jogging, yoga, or stretching increase blood flow to the brain and release endorphins, which enhance mood and cognitive clarity. Even a short 15-minute workout can make a difference. Mental exercises like puzzles or reading a stimulating book can also prime your brain for the day ahead. These activities engage your brain, improving memory, problem-solving skills, and overall mental agility. By combining physical and mental exercises, you create a holistic approach suitable for your needs to kick-starting your day.

Practicing mindfulness and meditation in the morning can help reduce stress and improve focus. Mindfulness involves paying attention to the present moment without judgment, which can be achieved through simple practices like focused breathing or body scan meditations. Start with just five minutes of mindfulness meditation each morning. Sit comfortably, close your eyes, and focus on your breath. If your mind wanders, gently bring your attention back to your breathing. Practicing this can help calm your mind, reduce anxiety, and set a positive tone for the rest of the day, and over time, you may be better able to manage stress and maintain focus on your tasks.

Journaling is another powerful tool to include in your morning routine. Writing down your thoughts, goals, and gratitude can promote a positive mindset and clarify your intentions for the day. Start by jotting down three things you're grateful for each morning. This practice shifts your focus from stressors to positive aspects of your life, enhancing your mood and cognitive flexibility.

Additionally, use your journal to outline your goals and plan your day. Writing down clear, achievable goals helps you stay organized and focused. Limit your daily goals to three essential actions that will move you closer to your larger objectives. Using this approach reduces cognitive load and ensures you prioritize tasks that truly matter.

Planning and organizing your day is the final component of a successful morning routine. Setting clear and attainable goals will help you stay focused and productive. Begin by determining the essential actions you must take today. Limit these to no more than three key tasks to avoid feeling overwhelmed. Break down larger tasks into smaller, manageable steps and prioritize them based on urgency and importance. By organizing your day this way, you create a roadmap that guides your actions and keeps you on track, enhancing productivity and reducing stress throughout the day.

Incorporating these elements into your morning routine can transform how you start your day, enhancing cognitive function and overall brain health. The key is to start small and gradually build your routine over time. Consistency is crucial to a sustainable outcome, so commit to your new habits and allow yourself the flexibility to adapt as needed. As you refine your morning routine, you'll likely feel more focused, energized, and ready to tackle whatever the day brings.

3.2 BRAIN TRAINING GAMES THAT WORK

Choosing suitable brain training games can be challenging, given the many options available. The key lies in discerning which games truly enhance cognitive abilities and which only stick to entertaining. Effective brain games should target specific cognitive skills such as problem-solving, memory, and processing speed. Look for games that offer progressively challenging levels, as this ensures continuous mental engagement. A good brain game will be enjoyable and push you to think critically and adapt to new problems. Games that require strategic thinking, pattern recognition, and quick decision-making are particularly beneficial. Avoid repetitive games that offer little variation, as they may not provide the cognitive stimulation needed for actual neuroplastic benefits.

Several games have been proven to improve cognitive functions effectively, including crossword puzzles, which challenge your vocabulary and problem-solving skills. They require you to think of words that fit a specific pattern, boosting your language and critical thinking abilities. Sudoku is another excellent option, as it focuses on numerical patterns and logic, advancing your problem-solving and memory skills. For a more interactive experience, consider computer-based applications like Lumosity and BrainHQ. These apps offer a variety of games designed to improve different cognitive skills, from memory to attention and processing speed. They adapt to your performance, ensuring you are constantly challenged at the right level. For beginners, games like Peak and Elevate are user-friendly and provide a good starting point for enhancing cognitive functions.

Integrating brain games into your daily routine doesn't have to be a tedious task. The goal is to make these activities seamless in your day without becoming monotonous or time-consuming. For instance, set aside a specific time each day for brain training, such as during your morning coffee or before bed, remembering that even 10 to 15 minutes daily can make a significant difference. To keep things interesting, rotate between different types of games. One day, you might focus on crossword puzzles, the next on Sudoku, and another on a memory game app. This variety ensures that you frequently challenge different areas of your brain, keeping it flexible and strong. Consider playing these games during breaks at work or while commuting, turning idle moments into opportunities for cognitive enhancement.

Tracking your progress is crucial for staying motivated and seeing tangible proof of your cognitive improvements. Many brain training apps offer built-in tracking features that monitor your performance over time. These features allow you to see how your skills improve, providing a sense of accomplishment and encouraging you to keep going. For more traditional games like crosswords and Sudoku, consider keeping a journal where you note your completion times and any difficulties you encounter. This practice helps you track your progress and provides insights into which areas you might need to focus on more. Additionally, setting specific goals, such as improving your puzzle completion time or advancing to a higher level in a brain training app, can provide clear milestones to strive for.

Incorporating brain training games into your daily life can be a highly effective way to enhance cognitive functions. By choosing the right games, integrating them smoothly into your routine, and tracking your progress, you can significantly improve problem-solving, memory, and processing speed. The benefits of these activities extend beyond mere entertainment, providing noticeable improvements in your cognitive health and overall mental agility.

3.3 TECHNIQUES FOR IMPROVING MEMORY RETENTION

Memory is a cornerstone of our cognitive abilities and improving it can profoundly affect our daily lives. One effective technique is the method of loci, also known as the memory palace. This ancient mnemonic device involves visualizing a familiar place and associating each piece of information you want to remember with a specific location. For example, suppose you're trying to memorize a grocery list. In that case, you might imagine walking through your house and placing each item in a different room. The loaf of bread could be on the kitchen counter, the carton of milk in the living room, and so forth. As you mentally walk through your house, these visualized locations help trigger the memory of each item.

Another powerful technique is chunking, which involves breaking down large amounts of information into smaller, manageable chunks. This is particularly useful for memorizing numbers or sequences. For instance, instead of trying to remember a long string of numbers like 149217762003, you can break it down into chunks: 1492, 1776, 2003. This method leverages the brain's natural tendency to find patterns, making it easier to recall the information later. Chunking can also be applied to text, such as breaking down a speech into key points or a long list into categories.

Mnemonic devices, such as acronyms and rhymes, are another effective way to boost memory retention. Acronyms are words formed from the first letters of a series of words, like using HOMES to remember the Great Lakes (Huron, Ontario, Michigan, Erie, Superior). Rhymes and songs can also aid memory by providing a rhythmic and melodic structure that makes information easier to recall. For example, many people remember the order of operations in mathematics (Parentheses, Exponents, Multiplication and Division, Addition and Subtraction) with the phrase "Please Excuse My Dear Aunt Sally."

Regular practice and repetition are crucial for strengthening memory pathways. Just as muscles grow stronger with regular exercise, neural connections in the brain become tougher with repeated use. Repetition helps solidify information in long-term memory, making it easier to retrieve when needed, which is why studying a little bit each day is more effective than cramming all at once. When learning new material, review it multiple times over several days or weeks. This spaced repetition technique ensures that the information moves from short-term to long-term memory, where it can be accessed more readily.

Applying these memory techniques in real-world contexts can significantly enhance your cognitive abilities. For example, if you're studying for an exam, use the loci method to create a mental map of the key concepts. Visualize each concept in a specific location within your memory palace, and mentally walk through it as you review. Chunking can help you remember complex procedures or large amounts of data for work-related tasks. Break down the information into smaller sections and focus on mastering each chunk before moving on to the next. Mnemonic devices can be handy for remembering names, dates, or technical terms. You can create acronyms or rhymes to help you recall the information quickly.

Lifestyle factors, including lack of sleep, poor diet, and chronic stress can all have a detrimental effect on memory retention and neuroplasticity. Sleep, in particular, is vital for memory consolidation, as it allows the brain to process and store information from the day. To ensure optimal brain function, it's crucial to aim for 7 to 9 hours of quality sleep each night. A balanced diet rich in omega-3 fatty acids, antioxidants, and vitamins can nourish the brain and enhance memory. Foods like fatty fish, berries, and leafy greens are especially beneficial. Chronic stress releases cortisol, a hormone that can damage the hippocampus, the brain region responsible for memory. Managing stress through mindfulness practices, regular exercise, and relaxation techniques can also improve memory retention.

Incorporating these memory-boosting techniques into your daily life can considerably improve your cognitive abilities. Whether studying for an exam, managing work tasks, or simply remembering where you left your keys, these strategies can help you retain and recall information more effectively. Practicing regularly and making healthy lifestyle choices can enhance your memory and unlock your brain's full potential.

3.4 STRATEGIES FOR OVERCOMING NEGATIVE THOUGHT PATTERNS

Understanding cognitive distortions is the first step in overcoming negative thought patterns. Cognitive distortions are biased ways of thinking about oneself and the world around you, often reinforcing negative emotions and making it difficult to see situations clearly and objectively. One common distortion is all-or-nothing thinking, where you see things in black and white, with no middle ground. For example, you might think, "If I fail this task, I'm a complete failure." Another is catastrophizing, where you expect the worst possible outcome. On the other hand, overgeneralization involves taking a single adverse event and viewing it as a never-ending pattern of defeat. By recognizing these distortions, you can begin to challenge and change them, paving the way for more balanced and accurate thinking.

Cognitive restructuring techniques are practical tools to help you identify, challenge, and replace negative thoughts with more posi- tive, realistic ones. One effective method is self-monitoring, where you keep a thought diary to track negative thoughts as they occur. Write down the situation, your thoughts, and the emotions you felt. Next, use questioning assumptions to challenge these thoughts and ask yourself if there is concrete evidence to support them or if they are based on assumptions. For instance, if you think, "I'll never be good at this," ask, "What evidence do I have that supports this thought?" Gathering evidence involves comparing facts that support or refute your beliefs. Perform a cost-benefit analysis to weigh the pros and cons of maintaining specific thought patterns. Finally, alternatives can be generated by creating positive affirmations and rational explanations to replace distortions. For example, replace "I always mess up" with "I made a mistake, but I can learn from it and improve."

Positive affirmations can rewire your thought patterns and contribute to more resilient neural pathways. When you repeatedly think positive thoughts, your brain strengthens those neural connections, making it easier to think positively in the future. Positive affirmations are simple, optimistic statements that you repeat to yourself to challenge and overcome self-sabotaging and negative thoughts. For example, you might say, "I am capable and strong," or "I can handle whatever comes my way." The key is to choose affirmations that resonate with you and repeat them consistently, especially during challenging times. Over time, these affirmations can help shift your mindset, making you more hopeful and resilient.

The long-term benefits of maintaining a positive outlook are overwhelming. Enhanced mood is one of the most immediate benefits, as positive thinking reduces stress and increases happiness. Better stress management is another significant advantage. When you approach challenges with a positive mindset, you're more likely to see them as opportunities for growth rather than insurmountable obstacles. This perspective can reduce the physiological effects of stress, such as high blood pressure and anxiety. Improved overall mental health is the ultimate benefit, as a positive outlook can decrease the risk of depression and anxiety, improve relationships, and increase life satisfaction. By cultivating a habit of positive thinking, you can create a more fulfilling and balanced life.

Interactive Element: Cognitive Restructuring Worksheet

To help you practice cognitive restructuring, consider using a worksheet to guide you through the process. Here's a simple template:

1. **Situation**: Describe the situation that triggered the negative thought.
2. **Negative Thought**: Write down the negative thought you had.
3. **Emotion**: Note the emotion you felt as a result of the thought.
4. **Evidence For**: List any evidence that supports the negative thought.
5. **Evidence Against**: List evidence that refutes the negative thought.
6. **Alternative Thought**: Create a more balanced, positive thought to replace the negative one.

Example:

1. **Situation**: Failed a test
2. **Negative Thought**: "I'm not smart enough to pass this course."
3. **Emotion**: Discouraged
4. **Evidence For**: "I did poorly on the test."
5. **Evidence Against**: "I've passed other tests in this course. I studied hard and understood the material."
6. **Alternative Thought**: "This was a tough test, but I can learn from my mistakes and do better next time."

By regularly filling out this worksheet, you can actively engage in cognitive restructuring and develop a more positive and realistic mindset.

3.5 BUILDING A PERSONALIZED NEUROPLASTICITY ROUTINE

Creating a personalized neuroplasticity routine begins with assessing your cognitive needs and setting realistic goals. Take a moment to reflect on areas where your mental abilities could improve. Are you looking to enhance memory, boost problem-solving skills, or reduce stress? Identifying your specific needs will help you tailor activities that target these areas. Write down your goals, making sure they are clear and achievable. For example, if you want to improve memory, your goal might be to remember names more easily or to retain information from books and articles. No matter what you want to accomplish, setting these goals provides direction and helps you focus on what matters most.

Customizing activities to match your interests, strengths, and weaknesses is crucial for keeping your neuroplasticity routine engaging and effective. If you enjoy reading, incorporate reading comprehension exercises or join a book club to stimulate your brain. Activities like dance, martial arts, or hiking can provide mental and physical stimulation for those who love physical activity. If you find puzzles intriguing, consider integrating various types of puzzles, from jigsaw to logic puzzles, into your routine. The idea is to choose activities you find enjoyable and challenging, ensuring you stay motivated and committed to your neuroplasticity routine. To help you get started, create a simple template that outlines your goals, preferred activities, and a weekly schedule, serving as a guide to stay on track.

Incorporating variety into your neuroplastic activities is vital for constantly challenging your brain and preventing plateauing. Just as your muscles need different exercises to strengthen, your brain benefits from diverse cognitive challenges. For instance, you might focus on memory exercises one day, problem-solving puzzles the next, and creative writing another day. This diversity keeps your routine interesting and stimulates different areas of your brain, promoting overall cognitive health. Think of it as a balanced diet for your brain, where each type of activity provides different nutrients that contribute to your mental welfare. Regularly updating your routine with new activities can help you discover new interests and strengths.

Monitoring your progress is essential for ensuring continued growth and satisfaction. Keep a journal or use a digital app to track your activities and note any improvements in your cognitive abilities. Write down what activities you did, how long you spent on them, and any observations about your performance. For example, you might notice that you're solving puzzles more quickly or that your memory has improved when recalling meeting details. These observations provide tangible proof of your progress and can be incredibly motivating.

Additionally, regularly reviewing and adjusting your goals as needed ensures that your routine aligns with your evolving needs and interests. If a particular activity no longer challenges you, consider increasing its difficulty or trying something new. This ongoing adjustment and evaluation keep your routine dynamic and effective.

Reflection Section: Personalized Neuroplasticity Routine Template

Try using this template as a guide to help you build your personalized routine. It will help you organize your goals, activities, and schedule, ensuring you have a clear plan.

1. Goals:

- Improve memory (e.g., remember names, retain information)
- Enhance problem-solving skills (e.g., faster puzzle-solving)
- Reduce stress (e.g., better emotional regulation)

2. Preferred Activities:

- Reading comprehension exercises
- Dance or martial arts
- Puzzles (jigsaw, logic)
- Creative writing

3. Weekly Schedule:

- Monday: Memory exercises (30 minutes)
- Tuesday: Dance class (1 hour)
- Wednesday: Puzzles (30 minutes)
- Thursday: Creative writing (30 minutes)
- Friday: Reading comprehension (30 minutes)
- Saturday: Hiking (2 hours)
- Sunday: Rest and reflection

By filling out this template, you create a systematized approach to your neuroplasticity routine. Adjust it as needed to keep it aligned with your goals and interests. This personalized plan will help you stay organized and challenge your brain meaningfully.

Building a personalized neuroplasticity routine involves understanding your cognitive needs, customizing activities to match your interests, incorporating variety, and monitoring your progress. This comprehensive approach ensures that your routine remains engaging, effective, and aligned with your goals. As you refine and adjust your routine, you'll be better equipped to enhance your cognitive abilities and overall mental wellness.

3.6 TEST YOUR KNOWLEDGE

As you reach the end of this chapter on practical applications of neuroplasticity, it's important to consolidate your understanding and ensure you're ready to implement these concepts into your daily life. The following quiz will help reinforce the critical concepts and practical applications discussed. Engaging with these questions will solidify your grasp on enhancing brain health and cognitive function through everyday practices.

Question 1: True or False: Regularly engaging in physical exercise can increase brain-derived neurotrophic factor (BDNF) levels, which supports the growth and differentiation of new neurons and synapses.

Question 2: Multiple Choice: Which of the following is a memory-boosting technique that involves visualizing a familiar place and associating each piece of information you want to remember with a specific location within it?

A) Chunking
B) Method of loci
C) Mnemonic devices
D) Positive affirmations

Question 3: True or False: Cognitive distortions are biased ways of thinking that can reinforce negative emotions and hinder neuro-plasticity.

Question 4: Multiple Choice: Which morning activity can help regulate your circadian rhythm and improve cognitive function by signaling to your brain that it's time to be alert?

A) Drinking a cup of coffee
B) Exposure to natural light
C) Checking emails
D) Watching TV

Question 5: True or False: Chunking involves breaking down large amounts of information into smaller, manageable pieces to make them easier to remember.

Question 6: Multiple Choice: What is the primary benefit of using positive affirmations regularly?

A) They provide entertainment
B) They rewire thought patterns and contribute to more resilient neural pathways
C) They improve physical health
D) They increase sleep quality

Question 7: True or False: Practicing mindfulness and meditation in the morning can help reduce stress and improve focus for the rest of the day.

Question 8: Multiple Choice: Which of the following is NOT a component of a personalized neuroplasticity routine?

A) Assessing personal cognitive needs and goals
B) Customizing activities to match interests and strengths
C) Avoiding variety in activities to maintain focus
D) Monitoring progress and adjusting the routine

Question 9: True or False: A balanced breakfast with protein, healthy fats, and complex carbohydrates supports sustained energy levels and provides necessary nutrients for brain function.

Question 10: Multiple Choice: Which cognitive restructuring technique involves keeping a thought diary to track negative thoughts and challenging them with evidence?

A) Positive affirmations
B) Self-monitoring
C) Chunking
D) Method of loci

Answers:

1. True
2. B) Method of loci
3. True
4. B) Exposure to natural light
5. True

6. B) They rewire thought patterns and contribute to more resilient neural pathways
7. True
8. C) Avoiding variety in activities to maintain focus
9. True
10. B) Self-monitoring

Reflecting on these questions helps ensure that you have a solid understanding of the practical applications of neuroplasticity. Each practice, from morning routines to memory techniques, contributes to a holistic approach to enhancing cognitive function and brain health. Integrating these strategies into your daily life reinforces your knowledge and actively supports your cognitive abilities. As you move forward, continue to explore and refine these practices, recognizing the profound impact they can have on your mental agility and resilience.

Next, we will explore how neuroplasticity impacts different age groups and offer strategies tailored to various stages of life to maximize cognitive health and brain function.

YOUR THOUGHTS MATTER—WE'D LOVE TO HEAR FROM YOU!

Thank you for taking the time to read *Neuroplasticity for Beginners*. As you continue exploring the transformative power of neuroplasticity, I hope the insights and examples have sparked new perspectives or helped answer some of your questions about how the brain can rewire itself.

If you're finding value in the book so far, I would greatly appreciate it if you could take a moment to share your thoughts by leaving a review. Your feedback is incredibly helpful for me as the author and helps other readers discover how understanding neuroplasticity can positively impact their lives.

Why Your Review is Important

Your review helps others decide whether this book is the right fit for them, whether they're just beginning to learn about neuroplasticity or seeking practical ways to apply it in their daily lives. Whether brief or detailed, every review contributes to spreading the word about the power of brain change.

How to Leave a Review

It's simple:

1. Head to the platform where you purchased the book, such as Amazon.
2. Find where you place orders (Returns & Orders is in the menu on Amazon).
3. Find your order of *Neuroplasticity for Beginners* and choose Write a Product Review.

What to Share in Your Review

Not sure where to start? Here are a few guiding questions:

- What insights or examples have resonated with you so far?
- Has the book changed how you view your brain's potential for growth?
- Are the concepts easy to understand, even for a beginner?

I sincerely value any feedback you're willing to provide, and I'm grateful that you're taking part in this journey of learning and discovery.

Thank you for being a part of this journey with me.

With gratitude,

- Hector J. Bordas, Author of *Neuroplasticity for Beginners*

CHAPTER FOUR
NEUROPLASTICITY ACROSS AGE GROUPS

Let's form a picture of a young child, eyes wide with curiosity, eagerly exploring their surroundings. Every new experience, from stacking blocks to hearing a bedtime story, is a building block in the architecture of their brain. This wondrous capability is neuroplasticity in action. Neuroplasticity isn't just a concept for adults trying to stave off cognitive decline or recover from injuries; instead, it's a fundamental aspect of early childhood development. In these formative years, the brain is extraordinarily malleable, shaped greatly by interactions, experiences, and the environment. Understanding how to enhance brain development in children through neuroplasticity is crucial, as these early years lay the groundwork for lifelong cognitive and emotional health.

4.1 ENHANCING BRAIN DEVELOPMENT IN CHILDREN THROUGH NEUROPLASTICITY

The foundation of early cognitive development is intricately linked with neuroplasticity, as the brain undergoes rapid growth during early childhood, and the neural pathways are highly receptive to new information. This period is characterized by the formation of synapses at an astonishing rate, which serves as the framework for future learning and cognitive abilities. The brain's architecture is built through repeated experiences and interactions, much like how a house is constructed brick by brick. For example, when a child learns to speak, their brain forms new connections that facilitate language processing and comprehension. These early experiences are critical because they establish the neural pathways the child uses throughout life. Thus, providing a stimulating and supportive environment during these formative years is essential for optimal brain development.

Activities that promote neuroplasticity in children are both diverse and engaging. Interactive play is one of the most effective ways to enhance neuroplasticity. Activities like building with blocks, solving puzzles, and playing dress-up stimulate different brain areas, fostering creativity, problem-solving skills, and fine motor coordination. Music lessons are another powerful tool. For example, learning to play an instrument involves auditory, visual, and motor skills, creating new neural connections and enhancing cognitive abilities. Language learning is equally beneficial. Introducing children to a second language early can significantly improve their brain's plasticity, as it involves complex cognitive processes like memory, listening, and speaking. Practical activities such as singing songs in different languages, reading bilingual books, and engaging in interactive language apps can make learning fun and effective.

The role of nutrition in children's brain development cannot be emphasized enough. Proper nutrition provides the essential nutrients required for ideal neural growth and function. Omega-3 fatty acids in foods like fish, flaxseeds, and walnuts are critical for brain development, as they help build cell membranes and support synaptic plasticity. Antioxidants in fruits and vegetables protect the brain from oxidative stress and support cognitive functions. Proteins, which supply the amino acids necessary for neurotransmitter production, are found in lean meats, eggs, and legumes.

Additionally, vitamins and minerals like iron, zinc, and magnesium play crucial roles in brain health. Iron is essential for oxygen transport to the brain, while zinc supports neurotransmitter functioning. Ensuring children have a balanced diet rich in these nutrients can significantly enhance their brain's plasticity and overall cognitive development.

Parental and educational influences are paramount in fostering a neuroplastic-friendly atmosphere for children. Parents play a vital role in shaping their children's brain development through their interactions and the environment they create. Engaging in activities like reading together, playing educational games, and encouraging curiosity can stimulate neural growth. Educational environments also play a crucial role, where schools and educators can enhance neuroplasticity by adopting teaching methods that encourage active learning and critical thinking. Incorporating hands-on activities, group projects, and problem-solving tasks into the curriculum can promote cognitive development. Moreover, creating an understanding and emotionally safe environment using techniques like positive reinforcement, encouragement, and nurturing relationships helps build a child's confidence and resilience, enhancing their brain's plasticity.

Interactive Element: Brain-Boosting Activities Checklist

To help parents and educators foster neuroplasticity in children, here is a checklist of brain-boosting activities that can be easily incorporated into daily routines:

▷ **Interactive Play:**

- Building with blocks or Legos.
- Solving age-appropriate puzzles.
- Engaging in imaginative play with costumes and props.

▷ **Music Lessons:**

- Learning to play a simple instrument like a keyboard or ukulele.
- Singing songs together and clapping to the rhythm.
- Listening to various genres of music and discussing the sounds.

▷ **Language Learning:**

- Reading bilingual storybooks.
- Using language learning apps designed for children.
- Playing language-based games like matching words to pictures.

▷ **Nutritional Support:**

- Including omega-3-rich foods like fish and flaxseeds in meals.
- Offering a variety of fruits and vegetables daily.

- Ensuring adequate protein intake through lean meats, eggs, and legumes.

▷ **Parental Interaction:**

- Reading together every day.
- Encouraging questions and exploring answers together.
- Playing educational games that promote critical thinking.

▷ **Educational Activities:**

- Participating in group projects and collaborative tasks.
- Engaging in hands-on science experiments.
- Encouraging problem-solving through games and activities.

By incorporating these activities and creating a supportive environment, parents and educators can significantly enhance children's neuroplasticity and cognitive development, laying a solid foundation for their future learning and growth.

4.2 NEUROPLASTICITY IN ADULTS: MAINTAINING COGNITIVE HEALTH

Many people believe that adult brains are fixed and incapable of growth. However, the reality is that adults can still form new neural connections, and this ongoing capacity for change is crucial for maintaining cognitive health. One compelling case study involved a group of middle-aged individuals participating in a six-month cognitive training program. The study, published in *Nature Neuroscience*, showed that participants exhibited significant improvements in memory, problem-solving skills, and even structural changes in the brain, such as increased gray matter density in regions associated with these functions. This evidence debunks the myth that adult brains cannot grow and underscores the importance of continuous mental stimulation.

Several lifestyle factors can significantly impact adult neuroplasticity. As discussed in Chapter 2, stress, lack of sleep, poor diet, a sedentary lifestyle, and substance abuse can all have detrimental effects on the brain's ability to form new connections. Chronic stress, for example, can lead to the release of cortisol. This hormone can damage the hippocampus, which is critical for memory and learning. Similarly, inadequate sleep disrupts the brain's ability to consolidate memories and repair itself. Poor dietary choices like excessive sugars and unhealthy fats can impair cognitive functions. At the same time, a lack of physical activity reduces the production of brain-derived neurotrophic factor (BDNF), a protein essential for neuroplasticity. Understanding these factors and actively working to mitigate them is critical for maintaining a healthy, adaptable brain.

Your professional environment and remote work settings offer numerous opportunities to enhance neuroplasticity. Engaging in problem-solving activities stimulates the brain's executive functions, promoting cognitive flexibility and resilience. Continuous learning, such as taking on new projects or acquiring new skills, keeps neural pathways active and adaptable. Collaboration with colleagues, whether through brainstorming sessions or team projects, fosters social interaction and cognitive engagement. Simple strategies to incorporate neuroplasticity practices into your professional life include:

- Setting aside time for focused problem-solving.
- Participating in professional development courses.
- Encouraging team collaboration on complex tasks.

Reflection Section: Workplace Neuroplasticity Practices

To help you implement the strategies above, here's a reflection exercise. Take a moment to think about your current professional environment. Identify one problem-solving activity you can engage in more frequently, one new skill you would like to learn, and one way to enhance collaboration with your colleagues. Write these down and set achievable goals for each. For example, you may spend 15 minutes daily on a complex problem-solving task, sign up for an online course about a new software tool, and suggest a weekly brainstorming session with your team. By setting these clear goals and actively working towards them, you can create a professional environment that supports and enhances your brain's neuroplasticity.

When you understand the capacity of the adult brain to grow and adapt and take conscious lifestyle and professional actions, you prioritize your cognitive health. Whether it's through strategic multitasking, continuous learning, or creating a neuroplastic-friendly workplace, the opportunities for enhancing your brain's plasticity is abundant and accessible.

Adults can adopt specific techniques and tools to further enhance neuroplasticity, such as strategic multitasking, which involves alternating between tasks that engage various cognitive functions. This practice improves efficiency and stimulates different brain areas, promoting neural growth. Complex problem-solving exercises, like puzzles, strategic games, or coding challenges, require the brain to think critically and adaptively, strengthening neural connections. Advanced learning commitments, like enrolling in online courses or attending workshops, provide new information and skills that keep the brain engaged and growing. Combined with a healthy lifestyle that includes regular exercise and a balanced diet, these activities can significantly enhance cognitive flexibility.

Here is an example of some daily practices you can incorporate into your schedule: Start your day with a short session of strategic multi-tasking, such as switching between a creative task like writing and an analytical task like data analysis. Incorporate complex problem-solving exercises into your breaks by solving a Sudoku puzzle or playing a strategic game like chess. Commit to advanced learning by setting aside weekly time to take an online course or read a book on a new subject. These small, manageable changes can make a big difference in maintaining and enhancing your brain's plasticity.

Reflecting on your lifestyle choices and making conscious adjustments can significantly improve your cognitive health. If you are frequently stressed, consider incorporating stress-reducing activities like mindfulness meditation or yoga into your routine. If sleep is an issue, establish a consistent sleep schedule and create a relaxing bedtime routine to improve sleep quality. Evaluate your diet and make small changes, such as adding more fruits and vegetables and reducing processed foods. Regular physical activity, even something as simple as a daily walk, can boost the production of BDNF and support neuroplasticity.

4.3 NEUROPLASTICITY FOR SENIORS: TECHNIQUES TO SLOW COGNITIVE DECLINE

As we age, our brains naturally undergo changes that can affect cognitive function. One of the common challenges older adults face is a slower processing speed, which can hinder the brain's ability to form new neural connections. While the rate of neuroplasticity does decline with age, it doesn't halt entirely. The efficiency and speed of synaptic changes may decrease, but the brain's capacity for growth and adaptation remains. Preventive measures taken earlier in life can help prolong these capabilities. Engaging in lifelong learning, maintaining a healthy diet, and staying physically active are all strategies that can support neuroplasticity well into older age. These proactive steps can mitigate the effects of aging on the brain, making it more resilient and adaptable.

Physical exercise plays a critical role in enhancing neuroplasticity in seniors, with suitable and stimulating activities significantly boosting brain function. Walking, for instance, is a simple yet effective exercise that increases blood flow to the brain, promoting the growth of new neurons and synapses. Tai Chi, a martial arts form involving slow, deliberate movements, is excellent for improving balance, coordination, and cognitive functioning. Research has shown that regular practice of Tai Chi can enhance memory and executive functioning in older adults. Swimming is another low-impact exercise that provides both physical and cognitive benefits. The rhythmic nature of swimming can have a meditative effect, reducing stress and promoting mental clarity. Incorporating these activities and others into a daily routine can help seniors maintain their cognitive health and provide neuroplastic improvement.

Social engagement is equally crucial for sustaining brain health in seniors. Interacting with others stimulates cognitive functions and provides emotional support, both vital for mental well-being. Community activities such as joining a book club, participating in group exercise classes, or attending local cultural events can foster social connections and stimulate the brain. Group therapies, such as reminiscence therapy, where seniors discuss past experiences, can also enhance cognitive function and emotional health. Online communities offer another avenue for social interaction, especially for those with mobility issues. Platforms like Facebook groups or online forums centered around shared interests can provide a sense of belonging and cognitive stimulation. Regular social engagement helps seniors stay mentally active, reducing the risk of cognitive decline.

Memory training programs and technologies designed for older adults can considerably boost neuroplasticity. Programs like Lumosity and BrainHQ offer cognitive exercises tailored to enhance memory, attention, and problem-solving skills. These programs adapt to the user's performance, ensuring the challenges remain engaging and effective. Another effective tool is mnemonic devices, which can aid in memory retention. Techniques such as the Method of Loci discussed previously, where individuals visualize placing items they want to remember in specific locations within a familiar space, can be particularly helpful. Technologies like virtual reality (VR) are also emerging as innovative tools for cognitive training. VR programs can create immersive environments that challenge the brain in new and interesting ways, promoting neuroplasticity. Regular participation in these memory training programs can help seniors maintain their cognitive functions and overall brain health.

Reflection Section: Memory Training Worksheet

To help seniors get started with memory training, here's a simple worksheet that can be used to practice mnemonic devices and other memory-enhancing techniques:

Memory Training Worksheet

1. Mnemonic Device Practice:

- Choose ten items you want to remember (e.g., grocery list).
- Use the Method of Loci: Visualize each item placed in a specific location within your home.

- Practice recalling the list by mentally walking through your home.

2. Daily Memory Exercise:

- Spend 10 minutes daily on a memory training app like Lumosity or BrainHQ.
- Track your progress and note any improvements in your memory and cognitive function.

3. Social Engagement Activity:

- Join a local club or online community that interests you.
- Participate in at least one weekly group activity to stay socially active.

4. Physical Exercise Routine:

- Incorporate a 30-minute walk, Tai Chi session, or swimming activity into your daily routine.
- Note any changes in your mood, energy levels, and cognitive sharpness.

By integrating these memory training techniques and activities into their daily lives, seniors can actively work to slow cognitive decline and enhance their brain's neuroplasticity. These practices improve memory, cognitive functions, and overall mental and emotional well-being.

4.4 INTERGENERATIONAL NEUROPLASTICITY: SHARING KNOWLEDGE ACROSS AGES

Imagine a classroom where children and seniors come together to learn, share stories, and engage in activities that stimulate their minds. This is the essence of cross-generational learning, where individuals from different age groups collaborate, fostering mutual growth and understanding. Intergenerational learning environments uniquely provide young and old participants with opportunities to enhance neuroplasticity together. For children, interacting with older adults can offer a wealth of knowledge and experience, helping to shape their cognitive and social skills. Conversely, seniors benefit from the mental stimulation and emotional uplift-ment of engaging with younger generations. These environments create a dynamic where both age groups can learn from each other, fostering a sense of community and shared purpose.

One inspiring example of intergenerational learning is the Experience Corps program, where older adults volunteer as tutors in elementary schools. This program has notably improved children's literacy and social skills while enhancing the older volunteers' cognitive functions. For instance, one participant named Joan, a retired teacher, found that tutoring children brought her joy and improved her memory and problem-solving abilities. On the other hand, the children benefited from Joan's patience and experience, which helped them grasp complex concepts more quickly. This reci-procal relationship exemplifies how intergenerational learning can lead to cognitive improvements on both ends of the age spectrum.

In another case study, the Downshall Primary School in East London implemented a program where older adults interacted with students to improve literacy and communication skills. The results were remarkable. Students not only showed improved reading abilities but also developed better interpersonal skills. The older adults reported feeling more connected and mentally stimulated, contributing to their overall wellness. These examples highlight the potential of intergenerational programs to create enriching learning experiences that benefit all participants. Such programs are not just about academic improvement; they also foster emotional and social growth, creating a more inclusive and supportive community.

Implementing intergenerational learning in communities, schools, and homes can be simple, with straightforward strategies making a substantial impact. Consider inviting seniors to share their life experiences during school history lessons, providing students with a living connection to the past. Community centers can organize weekly intergenerational activities such as art classes, gardening projects, or storytelling sessions. Families can encourage interactions between grandparents and grandchildren at home through shared hobbies like cooking, playing board games, or reading together. These activities stimulate the brain and strengthen familial bonds, creating an all-around supportive environment for cognitive growth.

The broader cultural and societal impacts of promoting intergenerational neuroplasticity are profound. One of the most significant benefits is the reduction of ageism. When younger and older generations interact frequently, it breaks down stereotypes and fosters mutual respect and understanding, leading to a more inclusive society where individuals are valued for their contributions regardless of age. Additionally, intergenerational learning can increase societal cohesion by creating opportunities for different age groups to collaborate and support each other. This sense of community can enhance overall health, as individuals feel more connected and less isolated.

Research has shown that intergenerational learning can boost children's social skills, increase school attendance, and deepen cultural and historical knowledge. For instance, in rural Australia, Aboriginal students who spent time with elders saw improvements in literacy, numeracy, confidence, and welfare. These benefits extend beyond the classroom, as students carry these skills and knowledge into their communities, fostering a sense of cultural pride and identity. Intergenerational learning offers older adults socio-emotional and health benefits, such as reducing feelings of loneliness and depression, improving cognitive function, and providing a renewed sense of purpose.

Strategies to promote intergenerational neuroplasticity can be tailored to fit various settings. Schools can create programs that pair students with older mentors for specific projects or subjects. Libraries and community centers can host intergenerational book clubs or technology workshops where seniors teach children new skills and vice versa. Local governments can support these initiatives by providing funding and resources to facilitate intergenerational activities. Encouraging businesses to adopt intergenerational practices, such as hiring older adults as part-time staff or mentors, can also contribute to a more inclusive workforce.

The cultural and societal impacts of intergenerational learning are far-reaching. By bringing together different age groups, we can create a more cohesive, respectful, and supportive society. These interactions enhance neuroplasticity and enrich our communities, making them stronger and more resilient. The benefits of intergenerational learning extend beyond the individuals involved, influencing broader cultural attitudes and societal structures. Through these efforts, we can foster a world where people of all ages are valued, respected, and given opportunities to contribute and grow.

4.5 LIFELONG LEARNING AS A TOOL FOR SUSTAINED NEUROPLASTICITY

Lifelong learning is the ongoing, voluntary, and self-motivated pursuit of knowledge for personal or professional reasons. It is not just about formal education; it encompasses many activities that stimulate the brain and foster continuous cognitive growth. This concept is critical for maintaining neuroplasticity, the brain's ability to reorganize itself by forming new neural connections. Engaging in lifelong learning keeps your brain active, adaptable, and capable of evolving with new experiences. It is an antidote to cognitive stagnation, ensuring your brain remains flexible and resilient as you age.

Numerous activities fall under the umbrella of lifelong learning, each offering unique benefits for brain health. Taking courses in unfamiliar subjects, whether online or in-person, exposes your brain to new information and challenges existing neural pathways. Creative arts, such as painting, writing, or playing a musical instrument, engage multiple brain regions simultaneously, enhancing cognitive flexibility. Learning a new language is another powerful way to stimulate the brain, as it involves complex processes like memorization, pronunciation, and comprehension. Reading and writing, whether for pleasure or education, keeps the brain engaged and improves cognitive functions. Even travel and participation in cultural events can serve as lifelong learning activities by exposing you to new environments and perspectives. Picking up new hobbies, such as gardening, cooking, or chess, can stimulate neuroplasticity by requiring the brain to learn and adapt to new tasks.

Practical suggestions for starting lifelong learning activities are plentiful and accessible, such as enrolling in an online course like astronomy or philosophy that sparks your interest. Many platforms offer free or low-cost courses, making this an easy entry point. You can also join a local art class or writing group to explore your creative side. Language learning apps such as Duolingo or Babbel can help you start learning a new language at your own pace. Set aside time each day for reading, whether a novel, a non-fiction book, or articles on topics that interest you. Plan a trip to a museum or a cultural festival in your area to immerse yourself in new experiences. If you prefer staying at home, consider picking up a new hobby like knitting, which is known to improve fine motor skills and cognitive functioning. The key is choosing activities that you find enjoyable and engaging, ensuring you remain motivated and committed.

While the benefits of lifelong learning are clear, several barriers can hinder your commitment to this practice. One of the most common obstacles is time constraints, as many people feel too busy with work, family, and other responsibilities to dedicate time to learning. However, incorporating learning into your daily routine can be more manageable than you think. For instance, you could listen to educational podcasts during your commute or read a chapter of a book before bed. Lack of resources can be another barrier, but the Internet provides plenty of free or affordable learning opportunities. Websites like Coursera, Khan Academy, and TED Talks provide high-quality educational content at no cost. Another common barrier is the need for more motivation or confidence, especially if you haven't engaged in formal learning for a long time. Starting with small, achievable goals can help build your confidence and motivate you. Set a timer for 10 minutes of learning each day and gradually increase it as you feel more comfortable.

The impact of lifelong learning on longevity and quality of life is well-documented, with studies showing that continuous learning can lead to a longer, healthier life. For example, a longitudinal study published in the *Journal of Epidemiology & Community Health* found that individuals who pursued lifelong learning had a lower risk of dementia and cognitive decline. Another study in the *British Medical Journal revealed* that people who engaged in educational activities throughout their lives had a higher life expectancy and better mental health. These findings highlight the importance of lifelong learning for cognitive health and overall well-being, as staying mentally active can enhance your quality of life, maintain mental sharpness, and lead to a fulfilling, intellectually rich life.

Incorporating lifelong learning into your daily routine can produce lasting benefits for your brain health. The opportunities for stimulating neuroplasticity are endless, whether through formal courses, creative pursuits, language learning, or new hobbies. Overcoming common barriers like time constraints and lack of resources is feasible with practical strategies and a commitment to prioritizing learning. The rewards of this commitment are significant, offering increased longevity, improved cognitive function, and a higher quality of life.

4.6 TEST YOUR KNOWLEDGE

Understanding and applying the principles of neuroplasticity across different age groups can be transformative. Let's reinforce what you've learned with a short quiz to ensure you can integrate these concepts into your life. This will help solidify your understanding and make the information more actionable.

Question 1: True or False: Older adults can experience significant improvements in cognitive function through regular physical exercise and social engagement.

Question 2: Multiple Choice: Which activity is particularly effective in promoting neuroplasticity in children?

A) Watching TV
B) Interactive play
C) Eating sugary snacks
D) Sitting quietly

Question 3: True or False: Lifelong learning only benefits cognitive health if started at a young age.

Question 4: Multiple Choice: What is a key benefit of cross-generational learning?

A) It makes children more competitive
B) It reduces ageism and fosters mutual respect
C) It isolates older adults
D) It focuses solely on academic learning

Question 5: True or False: Chronic stress does not impact adult neuroplasticity.

Question 6: Multiple Choice: Which nutrient is essential for optimal brain development in children?

A) Saturated fats
B) Omega-3 fatty acids
C) High-fructose corn syrup
D) Trans fats

Question 7: True or False: Engaging in complex problem-solving exercises can enhance neuroplasticity in adults.

Question 8: Multiple Choice: What is a common barrier to life-long learning?

A) Lack of interest

B) Time constraints

C) Overabundance of resources

D) Physical health

Question 9: True or False: Implementing intergenerational programs in schools can improve the cognitive functions of both students and seniors.

Question 10: Multiple Choice: Which strategy is recommended for maintaining cognitive health in seniors?

A) Avoiding social interactions

B) Engaging in group exercise classes

C) Consuming a diet high in sugars

D) Limiting physical activity

Answers:

1. True
2. B) Interactive play
3. False
4. B) It reduces ageism and fosters mutual respect
5. False
6. B) Omega-3 fatty acids
7. True
8. B) Time constraints
9. True
10. B) Engaging in group exercise classes

Reflect on your answers to understand where your strengths lie and which areas need more exploration. The goal is to test your knowledge and deepen your comprehension of how neuroplasticity principles can be applied in practical, everyday contexts.

Neuroplasticity is not confined to one stage of life; it spans the entire human lifespan. From enhancing brain development in children through engaging activities and proper nutrition to maintaining cognitive flexibility in adults and slowing cognitive decline in seniors, the principles of neuroplasticity can be a guiding light for lifelong cognitive health. Intergenerational learning environments and lifelong learning activities further enrich our understanding and application of neuroplasticity, fostering a society where every age group can thrive.

As you move forward, consider how these principles can be woven into your daily life. Whether it's through interactive play with children, continuous learning as an adult, or engaging in social activities as a senior, the opportunities to enhance brain health are abundant and accessible. Keep exploring, learning, and growing, and let the power of neuroplasticity lead you to a more vibrant, cognitively rich life.

In the next chapter, we will delve into practical applications and real-life examples to further illustrate how you can harness the power of neuroplasticity. Stay tuned for actionable insights that will empower you to take control of your cognitive health and unlock your brain's full potential.

CHAPTER FIVE

OVERCOMING NEUROLOGICAL CHALLENGES THROUGH NEUROPLASTICITY

You are sitting in a bustling café, the clinking of cups and the hum of conversation blend into the background. Across from you, a friend is sharing their struggle with anxiety, describing how it feels like a constant weight pressing down. They reveal they've tried countless methods to alleviate their symptoms, yet nothing seems to stick. You've seen this person light up with hope at the mention of a new therapy, only to watch that hope fade as the weeks pass. Now, imagine telling them that there's a way to change the very structure of their brain, to reshape it in a way that can lessen that weight.

This isn't a fantasy; it's the promise of neuroplasticity. Through targeted practices, you can rewire your brain to manage depression and anxiety effectively.

5.1 MANAGING DEPRESSION AND ANXIETY THROUGH NEUROPLASTIC TECHNIQUES

Cognitive Behavioral Therapy (CBT) is one of the most effective methods for treating depression and anxiety, leveraging the principles of neuroplasticity. In simple terms, CBT is talk therapy that helps you identify and change negative thought patterns and behaviors. It's like having a mental toolbox filled with strategies to challenge and replace those thoughts that drag you down. Studies have shown that CBT can significantly change brain structure and function. For example, research published in the journal *Translational Psychiatry* found that CBT can normalize excessive neural reactivity in the amygdala, a brain region associated with fear and anxiety. By engaging in CBT, you can reduce the gray matter volume in the amygdala, thereby decreasing your anticipatory anxiety and improving your overall mental health. This structural plasticity underscores how talking through and reframing your thoughts can greatly impact your brain's architecture.

Physical exercise is another powerful tool for managing symptoms of depression and anxiety. As discussed in Chapter 2, regular physical activity can alter the brain's stress response system, making you more resilient to stressors. Exercise increases the production of BDNF, a protein that supports the growth and differentiation of new neurons and synapses. This boost in BDNF helps to alleviate symptoms of depression and anxiety by promoting neurogenesis and enhancing brain plasticity. For instance, aerobic exercises like running, swimming, or cycling can elevate your mood by increasing dopamine and serotonin levels. These neurotransmitters play crucial roles in regulating mood and emotion. Regular exercise not only helps in the short term by providing a burst of endorphins but also offers long-term benefits for brain health, making it a cornerstone of any mental health strategy.

Mindfulness-Based Stress Reduction (MBSR) is another practical approach to managing anxiety and depression through neuroplasticity. MBSR is a structured program that combines mindfulness meditation, body awareness, and yoga to help you become more aware of the present moment. This practice has produced measurable changes in brain regions associated with memory, sense of self, empathy, and stress. A study by Massachusetts General Hospital and Harvard Medical School researchers, published in *Psychiatry Research: Neuroimaging,* found that participating in an eight-week MBSR program increased gray matter density in the hippocampus, which is important for learning and memory. Additionally, reductions in stress were correlated with decreased gray matter density in the amygdala, the region associated with anxiety and stress. These studies prove that practicing mindfulness can restructure your brain areas affected by these conditions, leading to greater well-being and improved quality of life.

In addition to specific therapies and exercises, making holistic lifestyle adjustments can significantly help manage depression and anxiety. Start by focusing on your daily habits, such as ensuring you sleep well each night, as sleep is vital for brain function and emotional regulation. Aim for 7 to 9 hours of quality sleep and establish a consistent sleep schedule by going to bed and waking up at the same time every day. Nutrition also plays a crucial role in mental health. Consume a balanced diet rich in omega-3 fatty acids, antioxidants, and vitamins. Foods like salmon, blueberries, and leafy greens can nourish your brain and improve cognitive functions. Avoid excessive sugar and processed foods, which can exacerbate symptoms of depression and anxiety.

Incorporating relaxation techniques into your daily routine can also help manage these conditions. Deep breathing, progressive muscle relaxation, and guided imagery can help activate the parasympathetic nervous system, reducing stress hormones and promoting relaxation. Additionally, engaging in social activities and maintaining strong social connections can provide emotional support and reduce feelings of isolation. Join a club, volunteer, or spend more time with friends and family. These interactions stimulate the release of oxytocin, a hormone that promotes bonding and reduces stress.

Reflection Section: Building a Mindfulness Routine

To help you get started with mindfulness practice, consider this simple routine:

- **Morning Mindfulness**: Begin your day with 5 to10 minutes of mindfulness meditation. Sit comfortably, close your eyes, and focus on your breath. If your mind wanders, gently bring your attention back to your breathing.
- **Body Scan**: In the evening, practice a body scan meditation for 10 to15 minutes. Lie down comfortably and mentally scan your body from head to toe, noticing any areas of tension and consciously relaxing them.
- **Mindful Eating**: Choose one meal daily to eat mindfully. Consider your food's colors, textures, and flavors. Eat slowly, savoring each bite.
- **Gratitude Journaling**: Write down three things you're grateful for before bed. This practice shifts your focus from stressors to positive aspects of your life, enhancing your mood and cognitive flexibility.

By incorporating these elements into your daily routine, you can create a structured approach to mindfulness that promotes relaxation and emotional wellness. This routine not only helps manage symptoms of depression and anxiety but also enhances your overall quality of life.

5.2 NEUROPLASTIC APPROACHES TO CHRONIC PAIN MANAGEMENT

What would you do if you woke up each day with a nagging pain that shadows every activity, making even simple tasks feel insurmountable? Chronic pain is not just a physical sensation; it's a complex interplay between your brain and body. Neuroplasticity offers a fascinating approach to understanding and managing chronic pain by altering how the brain perceives it. The brain's perception of pain is a learned response reinforced by repeated signaling from the body. Over time, this can create a persistent pain loop, even if the initial injury has healed. By leveraging neuroplasticity, you can retrain your brain to diminish these pain signals, effectively changing your experience of pain.

One effective method to use neuroplasticity for pain management is biofeedback. Biofeedback involves using electronic monitoring devices to gain awareness and control over physiological functions such as heart rate, muscle tension, and skin temperature. During a biofeedback session, sensors are attached to your skin, sending signals to a real-time monitor that displays your physiological responses. As you engage in relaxation exercises, you can see immediate feedback on the screen, allowing you to learn how to control these functions consciously. For example, practicing deep breathing or progressive muscle relaxation can lower your heart rate and reduce muscle tension. Over time, these techniques help retrain your brain to manage stress and pain more effectively. Biofeedback promotes relaxation and is beneficial for conditions like migraines, chronic pain, and anxiety.

Cognitive techniques such as Pain Reprocessing Therapy (PRT) also harness the principles of neuroplasticity to treat chronic pain. PRT is based on the understanding that chronic pain is often perpetuated by the brain's misinterpretation of normal sensory signals as painful. This therapy aims to rewire the brain's neural pathways to reinterpret these signals accurately. In simple terms, PRT involves identifying and challenging the beliefs and emotions that contribute to the pain experience. By reframing these beliefs and practicing new ways of thinking about pain, you can reduce its intensity and frequency. For instance, if you believe a specific movement will always cause pain, PRT helps you gradually test this belief and learn that the movement can be performed without pain. This cognitive shift alters the brain's pain processing pathways, reducing chronic pain symptoms.

Integrative practices that combine traditional and modern approaches can further support neuroplastic changes to alleviate chronic pain. Yoga, for example, is a practice that integrates physical postures, breath control, and meditation to promote overall well-being. Yoga has been shown to increase gray matter volume in brain regions associated with pain modulation, such as the insula and prefrontal cortex. Practicing yoga regularly can enhance your brain's ability to manage pain through improved body awareness and stress reduction. Additionally, targeted physical therapy exercises can help retrain the brain and body to move in ways that reduce pain and prevent further injury. A physical therapist can design a personalized exercise program for you to strengthen weak muscles, improve flexibility, and correct posture. These exercises address the physical aspects of pain and create new neural pathways that support pain-free movement.

Combining these integrative practices with cognitive techniques and biofeedback creates a holistic approach to chronic pain management. Here is an example of incorporating these practices into your routine: Start your day with a gentle yoga session to increase flexibility and reduce muscle tension. Throughout the day, you could use biofeedback techniques to monitor and control physiological responses to stress. Practicing PRT can help you reframe negative thoughts and beliefs about pain in the evening, reinforcing your brain's new neural pathways. This multifaceted approach addresses both the physical and psychological components of chronic pain, offering a comprehensive strategy for long-term relief.

Reflection Section: Biofeedback Practice

To help you get started with biofeedback, consider setting up a simple practice routine:

- **Choose a Biofeedback Device**: Select a device that measures physiological responses such as heart rate or muscle tension. Many wearable devices and apps are available for this purpose.
- **Set Up a Quiet Space**: Find a quiet, comfortable place to sit or lie down without distractions.
- **Practice Deep Breathing**: Begin with deep breathing exercises. Inhale slowly through your nose, hold for a few seconds and exhale slowly through your mouth. Watch the monitor to see how your heart rate or muscle tension responds.

- **Progressive Muscle Relaxation**: Gradually tense and relax different muscle groups, starting from your toes and working up to your head. Focus on the feedback from the monitor to learn how to control muscle tension.
- **Daily Routine**: Incorporate these practices into your daily routine, aiming for at least 10 to 15 minutes of daily biofeedback practice.

By consistently practicing these biofeedback techniques, you can develop greater awareness and control over your physiological responses, ultimately reducing the impact of chronic pain on your life.

5.3 COGNITIVE REHABILITATION FOR BRAIN INJURY PATIENTS

Picture waking up one day to find that everyday actions like tying your shoes or recalling a loved one's name have become monumental tasks. For many brain injury patients, this is a harsh reality. The path to recovery is paved with challenges, but the brain's remarkable ability to rewire itself offers a symbol of hope. Personalized cognitive rehabilitation plans are crucial, as they target specific brain areas affected by the injury and are tailored to address individual cognitive functions that need improvement. For example, if a patient has sustained damage to the frontal lobe, which is responsible for decision-making and problem-solving, the rehabilitation plan would include exercises designed to enhance these abilities. This targeted approach ensures that each patient receives the appropriate interventions to maximize their recovery potential.

Therapeutic exercises form the backbone of cognitive rehabilitation, designed to enhance memory, attention, and problem-solving skills.

For memory improvement, exercises include recalling a list of words after a short period or using mnemonics to remember information. Attention can be sharpened through activities that require sustained focus, such as sorting cards based on different criteria or playing attention-enhancing games. Problem-solving skills can be honed with puzzles, strategy games, and real-life scenarios that require critical thinking. For example, a patient might be asked to plan a small event, considering all the steps and resources needed. These exercises stimulate the brain and create new neural pathways, fostering cognitive resilience and adaptability.

Professional support is essential in cognitive rehabilitation, with neuropsychologists, occupational therapists, and other specialists offering the expertise and guidance needed for effective neuroplastic recovery. Neuropsychologists assess cognitive function and design customized rehabilitation programs that target specific deficits. Occupational therapists help patients relearn daily activities and develop strategies to compensate for lost functions. Speech therapists might work with patients who have language impairments, using techniques to improve communication skills. This multidisciplinary approach ensures that patients receive comprehensive care, addressing all aspects of their cognitive health. These professionals regularly assess and adjust the rehabilitation plan to ensure that the interventions remain effective and aligned with the patient's progress.

Success stories in cognitive rehabilitation serve as powerful motivators, showcasing the transformative potential of personalized neuroplasticity interventions. Take the case of John, a 45-year-old man who suffered a traumatic brain injury in a car accident. Initially, John struggled with basic tasks like remembering his children's names and following simple instructions. His cognitive rehabilitation plan included memory exercises, problem-solving activities, and physical therapy to improve coordination. John made remarkable progress with the support of a dedicated team of professionals. Within six months, he regained much of his cognitive function, returned to work, and even took up a new hobby—woodworking. Stories like John's highlight the incredible resilience of the human brain and the overwhelming impact of targeted rehabilitation.

Another incredible story is of Maria, a young woman who suffered a stroke that left her partially paralyzed and struggling with speech. Her rehabilitation journey was daunting, but with a personalized plan that included speech therapy, cognitive exercises, and physical therapy, Maria made remarkable strides. She practiced word recall exercises, engaged in activities that stimulated her problem-solving skills, and worked tirelessly on her physical rehabilitation. Over time, Maria regained her ability to speak fluently and move independently. Her story is a testament to the power of neuroplasticity and the importance of a comprehensive, individualized approach to rehabilitation.

David is one more inspiring example, a retired teacher who experienced a severe brain injury after a fall. David's initial prognosis was grim, with doctors predicting limited recovery. However, his personalized rehabilitation plan focused on enhancing his cognitive functions through targeted exercises and activities. David's plan included daily memory tasks, attention-enhancing games, and problem-solving challenges. With the unwavering support of his rehabilitation team, David not only regained his cognitive abilities but started mentoring younger teachers, sharing his experiences and insights. His journey underscores the critical role of specialized support and the potential for extraordinary recovery, even in seemingly dire circumstances.

Interactive Element: Personalized Cognitive Rehabilitation Plan Template

To help you understand the structure of a personalized cognitive rehabilitation plan, here's a simple template:

- **Assessment**: Detailed evaluation of cognitive deficits and strengths.
- **Goals**: Specific, measurable objectives tailored to the patient's needs.
- **Therapeutic Exercises**:

  - **Memory**: Word recall tasks, mnemonic strategies.
  - **Attention**: Sorting activities and attention-enhancing games.
  - **Problem-solving**: Puzzles, strategic planning scenarios.

- **Professional Support**: Regular sessions with neuropsychologists, occupational therapists, and speech therapists.
- **Progress Monitoring**: Regular assessments and adjustments to the plan based on patient progress.

Following this template, professionals can create comprehensive and effective rehabilitation plans catering to each patient's unique needs. This approach maximizes recovery potential and provides a structured pathway for cognitive improvement.

The power of neuroplasticity in cognitive rehabilitation is nothing short of miraculous. Patients can regain significant functionality and improve their quality of life through personalized plans, targeted exercises, professional support, and inspiring success stories. The recovery journey may be challenging, but with the right interventions and unwavering determination, the brain's capacity for change and adaptation can lead to impressive transformations.

5.4 ADHD AND NEUROPLASTICITY: STRATEGIES FOR SUCCESS

Behavioral interventions have shown significant promise in modifying the neural pathways associated with ADHD, leading to improvements in concentration and behavior. These interventions aim to reshape the brain's response to stimuli, helping individuals develop better self-regulation skills. One effective strategy is using positive reinforcement, where desirable behaviors are rewarded to encourage their recurrence. For example, a child with ADHD might receive a sticker for completing a task or following instructions, which can later be exchanged for a larger reward. This method leverages the brain's reward system, stimulating the release of dopamine, a neurotransmitter crucial for motivation and learning. Additionally, breaking tasks into smaller, manageable steps can help reduce the overwhelming feeling often accompanying larger projects. Teachers and parents can further aid by implementing structured routines and clear expectations to provide a consistent environment, which helps stabilize the brain's activity levels and enhances focus.

The impact of diet on brain health is particularly important for individuals with ADHD, as certain nutrients can support neuroplasticity and improve cognitive function. Omega-3 fatty acids, found in fish like salmon and sardines and in flaxseeds and walnuts, are essential for brain development and function. These fatty acids help maintain the fluidity of cell membranes, facilitating better communication between neurons. Studies have shown that children with ADHD often have lower levels of omega-3 fatty acids, and supplementation can lead to improvements in attention and behavior. A diet rich in fruits, vegetables, and whole grains also provides antioxidants and other nutrients that protect the brain from oxidative stress and inflammation. Conversely, reducing the intake of processed foods and sugars can prevent blood sugar spikes and crashes that exacerbate ADHD symptoms. Encouraging a balanced diet with adequate hydration can create a more stable internal environment, supporting overall brain health and enhancing neuroplasticity.

Exercise has been identified as a powerful tool in mitigating ADHD symptoms and enhancing cognitive function through neuroplastic changes. Physical activity boosts neurotransmitters such as dopamine, norepinephrine, and serotonin, which are crucial for attention and mood regulation. Aerobic exercises like running, swimming, and cycling are especially effective in increasing these levels. For example, a study published in the *Journal of Attention Disorders* found that children who participated in regular aerobic exercise showed significant improvements in attention, memory, and executive function. Exercise also promotes the release of BDNF, which supports the growth and differentiation of new neurons and synapses. Schools and parents can incorporate more physical activity into daily routines, such as short exercise breaks between lessons or family walks in the evening. These activities improve mood, focus, and long-term brain health.

Mindfulness and attention training are additional strategies that can help rewire the brain and improve symptoms of ADHD. Mindfulness practices involve paying attention to the present moment without judgment, which can help individuals with ADHD develop greater self-awareness and emotional regulation. Techniques like mindful breathing, body scans, and focused attention exercises can be incorporated into daily routines. For example, starting the day with a five-minute mindfulness meditation can set a calm and focused tone for the day. Research has shown that mindfulness practices can lead to structural changes in the brain, such as increased gray matter density in areas associated with attention and self-regulation. Attention training exercises, such as playing memory games or practicing sustained attention tasks, can also help strengthen the brain's ability to focus. These exercises challenge the brain to maintain attention over longer periods, gradually improving its capacity for sustained focus. Schools can assist students by introducing mindfulness programs and attention training exercises into the curriculum, providing students with tools to enhance their concentration and emotional resilience.

By integrating these behavioral interventions, nutritional strategies, exercise routines, and mindfulness practices, individuals with ADHD can experience improvements in their cognitive functioning and wellness. These approaches help manage symptoms and leverage the brain's natural ability to adapt and grow, fostering long-term neuroplastic changes that support better attention, behavior, and emotional regulation.

5.5 TEST YOUR KNOWLEDGE

After absorbing the detailed insights about managing depression and anxiety, chronic pain management, cognitive rehabilitation for brain injury, and strategies for addressing ADHD, it's time to reinforce what you've learned. This quiz will help you review critical concepts and practical applications, ensuring you can apply neuro-plasticity principles in your daily life.

Quiz: Understanding Neuroplastic Approaches

Question 1: True or False: Biofeedback can help individuals control physiological functions, such as heart rate and muscle tension, to manage chronic pain effectively.

Question 2: Multiple Choice: Which technique is used in cognitive rehabilitation to improve memory and attention in brain injury patients?

A) Aerobic exercise
B) Mindfulness meditation
C) Word recall tasks
D) Positive affirmations

Question 3: True or False: Behavioral interventions for ADHD can modify neural pathways, leading to improved concentration and behavior.

Question 4: Multiple Choice: What is a key nutrient that supports brain health and can help mitigate ADHD symptoms?

A) Omega-3 fatty acids
B) High-fructose corn syrup
C) Trans fats
D) Saturated fats

Question 5: True or False: Physical exercise increases levels of neurotransmitters like dopamine and serotonin, which play crucial roles in regulating mood and attention.

Question 6: Multiple Choice: Which cognitive technique involves reframing beliefs and practicing new ways of thinking about pain to reduce its intensity?

A) Biofeedback
B) Pain Reprocessing Therapy (PRT)
C) Cognitive Behavioral Therapy (CBT)
D) Mindfulness-Based Stress Reduction (MBSR)

Question 7: True or False: Integrative practices like yoga and targeted physical therapy can support neuroplastic changes that alleviate chronic pain.

Question 8: Multiple Choice: What role do neuropsychologists play in cognitive rehabilitation for brain injury patients?

A) Assessing cognitive function and designing customized rehabilitation programs
B) Providing physical exercise routines
C) Teaching mindfulness meditation
D) Recommending dietary supplements

Question 9: True or False: Mindfulness practices can lead to structural changes in the brain, such as increased gray matter density in areas associated with attention and self-regulation.

Question 10: Multiple Choice: Which approach combines physical postures, breath control, and meditation to promote overall well-being and manage chronic pain?

A) Cognitive Behavioral Therapy (CBT)
B) Mindfulness-Based Stress Reduction (MBSR)
C) Yoga

D) Biofeedback

Answers:

1. True
2. C) Word recall tasks
3. True
4. A) Omega-3 fatty acids
5. True
6. B) Pain Reprocessing Therapy (PRT)
7. True
8. A) Assessing cognitive function and designing customized rehabilitation programs
9. True
10. C) Yoga

Reflecting on these questions helps ensure that you have a solid understanding of the practical applications of neuroplasticity. Each practice, from managing depression and anxiety to addressing ADHD, contributes to a holistic approach to enhancing cognitive function and brain health. Integrating these strategies into your daily life, reinforces your knowledge and actively participates in your mental health.

This chapter has provided various neuroplastic techniques and strategies to manage neurological challenges. From cognitive behavioral therapy to biofeedback, personalized cognitive rehabilitation plans to behavioral interventions for ADHD, each approach leverages the brain's remarkable ability to adapt and grow. Embracing these methods can significantly improve mental and physical health, enhancing one's overall quality of life.

The next chapter will explore how creating a neuroplastic-friendly environment can further support your brain health journey. Stay tuned for actionable insights on designing spaces, social interactions, and educational systems that promote neuroplasticity.

CHAPTER SIX

CREATING A NEUROPLASTIC-FRIENDLY ENVIRONMENT

Have you ever walked into a room that feels like a sanctuary? The soft glow of natural light fills the space, the scent of fresh greenery invigorates your senses, and a water fountain's gentle hum creates a calm atmosphere. You feel your stress melting away, your mind becoming clear and focused. This isn't just a dream; it's the reality that neuro-architecture seeks to create. Neuro-architecture is an emerging field that merges neuroscience and architecture to design spaces that enhance well-being and cognitive function. Learning and applying its principles allows you to transform your living environment into a haven for your brain.

Neuro-architecture integrates various elements from neuroscience, architecture, physiology, and psychology to create spaces catering to human wellness's four pillars: physical, intellectual, emotional, and social. This multidisciplinary approach recognizes that our brain responds to environmental stimuli in ways that significantly impact our emotions, memory, decision-making, and overall behavior. For instance, studies have shown that symmetrical forms and curvilinear designs can enhance memory and perception. At the same time, high ceiling heights can promote creativity and positive emotions. By leveraging these insights, you can create environments that support and improve your brain's plasticity.

One of the most influential elements in a neuroplastic-friendly environment is natural lighting. Natural light regulates circadian rhythms, which are crucial for maintaining a healthy sleep-wake cycle. Exposure to natural light during the day can boost mood, increase alertness, and improve cognitive functions. To add more natural light to your life, position your workspace or living area near windows, using light, sheer curtains to allow sunlight to filter in while reducing glare. Additionally, incorporating mirrors can help reflect light throughout the room, creating a brighter, more inviting space. For those darker corners, opt for full-spectrum light bulbs that mimic natural daylight, supporting your brain's need for light even in the absence of windows.

Noise control is another critical aspect of creating a brain-healthy environment. Excessive noise can increase stress levels, reduce concentration, and impair mental functioning. To mitigate noise, use soft furnishings like rugs, curtains, and cushions to absorb sound and reduce echo. If you live in a particularly noisy area, consider installing soundproof windows or using white noise machines to mask disruptive sounds. Incorporating elements like water fountains or gentle background music can also create a calming auditory environment, helping to maintain focus and reduce stress.

Integrating nature into your living space can positively affect your mental well-being and cognitive abilities. Known as biophilic design, this approach emphasizes the connection between humans and nature, promoting environments that include natural elements. Adding indoor plants improves air quality, reduces stress, and boosts mood. Choose low-maintenance plants like snake plants or peace lilies and place them in areas where you spend the most time. Additionally, consider incorporating natural materials like wood and stone into your décor. Studies have shown that natural materials can lower heart rate and promote a sense of calm, contributing to a more relaxing and brain-friendly environment.

The layout and design of your home can considerably impact your psychological wellness. So, consider creating distinct zones within your living space to promote relaxation, concentration, and learning. Designate specific areas for different activities, such as a quiet reading nook, a dedicated workspace, and a relaxation area. Keep your workspace clutter-free and organized; a tidy environment can enhance focus and productivity. Use shelves, bins, and trays to keep items in place, reducing visual distractions. In your relaxation area, try incorporating elements like comfortable seating, soft lighting, and soothing colors to create a haven where you can unwind and recharge.

A fascinating case study illustrating the impact of architectural changes on mental health is the redesign of a high-stress office environment. Employees at a tech company reported high levels of stress and burnout, prompting the management to consult with experts in neuro-architecture.

The redesign included:

- The integration of natural light.
- Biophilic elements like indoor plants and water features.
- Quiet zones for focused work.

Post-renovation surveys revealed a significant reduction in stress levels, improved concentration, and increased job satisfaction among employees. This example underscores the potential of thoughtfully designed spaces to enhance cognitive functioning and overall well-being.

By understanding and applying neuro-architecture principles, you can create a living environment that supports your brain's health and plasticity. From maximizing natural light and controlling noise pollution to integrating nature and carefully designing your space, these elements promote a sense of calm, focus, and overall well-ness. As you make these changes, you'll likely find that your home becomes more than just a place to live—it becomes a sanctuary for your mind.

Reflection Section: Designing Your Neuroplastic Sanctuary

Take a moment to assess your current living environment. Are there areas that feel particularly calming or stressful? Make a list of changes you can implement to create a more neuroplastic-friendly space. Consider elements like lighting, noise control, and nature integration. Start with small changes, such as adding a plant to your workspace or repositioning your furniture to maximize natural light. Reflect on how these adjustments impact your mood, focus, and overall health.

6.1 THE IMPACT OF SOCIAL INTERACTIONS ON NEUROPLASTICITY

Picture yourself at a lively community center, surrounded by friends and family, where laughter, shared stories, and warm connections fill the air, leaving you joyful and energized. This isn't just a pleasant experience; it's a powerful boost to your brain's health. Social interactions are vital in neuroplasticity, profoundly influencing our brain's ability to adapt and thrive. Engaging with others stimulates cognitive functions, enhances emotional resilience, and fosters good health. Social connectivity is akin to a workout for the brain, challenging it to process information, interpret emotions, and respond dynamically.

When you interact with others, your brain releases neurotransmitters like dopamine and oxytocin, which are essential for bonding and emotional regulation. These chemicals help to strengthen neural connections, making social interactions a natural and enjoyable way to promote neuroplasticity. Engaging in meaningful conversations, participating in group activities, and maintaining close relationships can all contribute to a healthier, more adaptable brain. Social support acts as a buffer against stress, which is known to negatively impact neuroplasticity by damaging the hippocampus and prefrontal cortex. By fostering strong social connections, you create a protective environment for your brain, enhancing its resilience and capacity for growth.

On the flip side, loneliness and social isolation can have detrimental effects on neuroplasticity. Recent studies have shown that prolonged isolation can lead to a decline in cognitive functions, increased stress levels, and even structural changes in the brain. For instance, chronic loneliness has been linked to reduced gray matter volume in areas associated with social cognition and emotional regulation, which can result in difficulties with memory, attention, and problem-solving. Without social stimuli, the brain becomes less flexible and more susceptible to the harmful effects of stress, highlighting the importance of social interactions for maintaining cognitive health and overall happiness.

Improving your social interactions doesn't necessarily require a complete lifestyle overhaul; simply start by engaging in activities that interest you and naturally involve others. Joining clubs or groups that align with your hobbies can be a great way to meet new people and build connections. Whether it's a book club, a sports team, or a gardening group, these settings provide opportunities for meaningful interactions and shared experiences. Volunteering is another excellent way to enhance social connectivity. It allows you to contribute to your community and introduces you to like-minded individuals who share your values and interests. You can find local volunteer opportunities at community centers, schools, or non-profits.

For those who find it challenging to meet new people or maintain social connections, digital tools can be a valuable resource. Social media platforms, online forums, and virtual meetups can help you stay connected with friends and family, regardless of geographical barriers. These digital spaces offer a convenient way to engage in conversations, share experiences, and participate in group activities. For individuals with mobility issues or those living in remote areas, digital socialization can be a lifeline, providing a sense of community and belonging. Platforms like Zoom, Skype, and FaceTime make it easy to have face-to-face interactions, even when physical proximity isn't possible.

Incorporating social interactions into your daily routine can also be as simple as making small changes to your habits. Set aside time weekly to call or meet up with friends and family. Engage in casual conversations with neighbors or colleagues. Attend community events or workshops that interest you. These small steps can significantly affect your social connectivity and, consequently, your brain health. Remember, the goal is to create meaningful connections that enrich your life and stimulate your brain.

Practical Tips for Enhancing Social Interactions

1. **Join Local Clubs or Groups**: Find clubs or groups that align with your interests, such as a book club, sports team, or hobby group.
2. **Volunteer**: Look for volunteer opportunities in your community to meet like-minded individuals and contribute to a cause.
3. **Use Digital Tools**: Utilize social media, online forums, and virtual meetups to stay connected with friends and family.
4. **Schedule Regular Interactions**: Set aside time weekly to call or meet with loved ones.
5. **Engage in Casual Conversations**: In your daily life, try to interact with neighbors, colleagues, and community members.

Incorporating these strategies into your routine can enhance social interactions, support your brain's health, and promote neuro-plasticity.

6.2 EDUCATIONAL SYSTEMS AND NEUROPLASTICITY: EVOLVING APPROACHES

Please close your eyes and imagine sitting in a classroom where every student is fully engaged, their eyes wide with curiosity and minds buzzing with excitement. This isn't just a teacher's dream; it's a reality that can be achieved by integrating neuroplastic principles into educational curriculum design. By recognizing that every student's brain is unique and capable of change, we can create learning environments that cater to diverse learning styles and promote brain plasticity. This means moving away from one-size-fits-all approaches and embracing methods that adapt to individual needs. For example, incorporating visual, auditory, and kinesthetic learning activities can help ensure that each student's brain is engaged in ways that resonate most effectively with them. This approach makes learning more enjoyable and strengthens neural pathways, enhancing memory and understanding.

Innovative teaching methods can significantly enhance neuroplasticity in students. Project-based learning, for instance, immerses students in complex, real-world problems that require critical thinking, collaboration, and creativity. This method engages multiple brain regions, fostering the development of robust neural networks. Take, for instance, a science class where students are tasked with designing a sustainable garden. They must research plants, understand soil chemistry, and apply mathematical principles to lay out the garden. This hands-on approach makes learning tangible and memorable, reinforcing neural connections.

Similarly, flipped classrooms, where students review lecture material at home and engage in interactive classroom activities, allow for deeper understanding and application of knowledge. Experiential learning, which involves learning through reflection on doing, can also be a powerful tool. Whether a field trip to a historical site or a business scenario simulation, these experiences make abstract concepts concrete, facilitating long-lasting neural changes.

Lifelong learning programs are another crucial aspect of promoting neuroplasticity. These programs encourage continuous education and brain training beyond the traditional school years, acknowledging that the brain remains plastic throughout life. Adult education courses, community workshops, and online learning platforms allow individuals to acquire new skills, explore interests, and stay mentally active. For example, a local community center might offer language classes, art workshops, or technology training sessions catering to diverse interests and cognitive needs. By participating in these programs, adults can keep their brains engaged, fostering neuroplasticity and enhancing mental functions. This approach benefits individuals and contributes to a more knowledgeable and adaptable society.

Case studies in educational reform demonstrate the transformative power of neuroplastic-friendly approaches. Take the example of a school district that implemented a comprehensive neuroplasticity-based curriculum. The curriculum included project-based learning, flipped classrooms, and experiential activities, all designed to engage different learning styles and promote brain plasticity. Over time, teachers observed significant improvements in student engagement, understanding, and material retention. Standardized test scores rose, but more importantly, students displayed a greater love for learning and an increased ability to think critically and solve problems.

Another example is a university that introduced lifelong learning programs for its alumni. These programs offered courses in various subjects, from creative writing to computer programming, encouraging graduates to continue their intellectual growth. Participants reported enhanced cognitive functions, greater job satisfaction, and improved mental well-being, illustrating the long-term benefits of continuous education.

Integrating neuroplastic principles in educational systems is not just a theoretical ideal; it has practical and measurable outcomes. By designing curricula that cater to diverse learning styles, employing innovative teaching methods, and fostering lifelong learning, we can create environments that support and enhance brain plasticity. This approach improves academic performance and equips individuals with the cognitive tools they need to navigate an ever-changing world. As we continue to understand and apply the principles of neuroplasticity, the potential for educational reform becomes boundless, promising a future where learning is dynamic, inclusive, and transformative.

6.3 CORPORATE WELLNESS PROGRAMS: PROMOTING NEUROPLASTICITY AT WORK

Now, let's step into a workplace set up to boost our mental well-being and help you grow cognitively. More and more companies are rethinking their workspaces to promote better mental health and cognitive flexibility, understanding how much the environment influences brain function.

Open spaces that encourage movement and interaction, relaxation zones equipped with comfortable seating and calming decor, and incorporating natural elements like plants and water features are becoming increasingly common. These design choices are not just about aesthetics; they are grounded in the understanding that our surroundings can drastically impact our brain's plasticity. For instance, open spaces facilitate spontaneous communication and collaboration, stimulating creative thinking and problem-solving. Relaxation zones provide a quiet retreat from the hustle and bustle, allowing employees to recharge and return to tasks with renewed focus. Integrating nature into the workspace has been shown to reduce stress and enhance wellness, making it easier for the brain to adapt and grow.

Corporate programs enhancing mental health and neuroplasticity are becoming a cornerstone of workplace wellness initiatives. Workshops on stress management teach employees techniques to handle pressure effectively, reducing the negative impact of chronic stress on the brain. Mindfulness sessions, often held during lunch breaks or as part of the daily schedule, encourage employees to practice mindfulness meditation, increasing gray matter density in brain regions associated with attention and emotional regulation. Cognitive flexibility training, which includes exercises designed to improve mental agility and adaptability, helps employees stay sharp and responsive in a fast-paced work environment. These programs support individual mental health and contribute to a more dynamic and innovative workplace culture.

The benefits of promoting neuroplasticity in the workplace extend to both employers and employees. For employers, a workforce with enhanced cognitive flexibility and emotional resilience translates to increased productivity and creativity. Employees who feel mentally supported are more likely to be engaged and satisfied with their jobs, leading to higher retention rates and reduced recruitment costs. Moreover, focusing on mental health can lower healthcare costs, as employees are better equipped to manage stress and avoid burnout. The benefits for employees are equally beneficial, as participating in neuroplasticity programs can improve mental clarity, problem-solving skills, and provide a greater sense of contentment. This holistic approach to workplace wellness creates a positive feedback loop, where a supportive environment fosters a healthier, more productive workforce, contributing to the organization's overall success.

Implementing effective neuroplasticity-promoting wellness programs requires a strategic approach. Companies can begin by gathering employee feedback to understand their needs and preferences through surveys, focus groups, or suggestion boxes. Tailored health interventions that address specific areas of concern, such as stress management or cognitive training, are more likely to be effective and well-received. Providing various options allows employees to choose the activities that best fit their interests and schedules, increasing participation and engagement. Regularly evaluating the programs and soliciting feedback ensures they remain relevant and effective. For example, a company could start with a pilot program offering weekly mindfulness sessions and quarterly cognitive flexibility workshops, then gather participant feedback after a few months to adjust the offerings based on their experiences and suggestions.

To guide employers through the implementation process, consider these steps. Begin by assessing the current state of employee wellness through surveys or health assessments. Use this data to identify key areas for improvement and develop a wellness strategy that includes specific goals and metrics for success. Next, choose a variety of programs and activities that align with the identified needs, such as mindfulness training, stress management workshops, and cognitive exercises. Communicate the availability and benefits of these programs clearly to all employees, emphasizing the company's commitment to their well-being. Encourage participation by offering incentives, such as wellness rewards or extra break time. Finally, set up a system for ongoing evaluation and feedback, regularly reviewing program effectiveness and making adjustments to ensure they continue to meet the workforce's needs.

Creating a workplace that promotes neuroplasticity is not just about implementing programs; it's about fostering a culture that values mental health and continuous growth. When employees feel supported and empowered to take charge of their mental health, they are more likely to thrive personally and professionally. By integrating neuroplasticity principles into the workplace, companies can create environments where innovation and productivity flourish, and employees feel valued and equipped to reach their full potential.

6.4 THE ROLE OF PUBLIC POLICY IN SUPPORTING NEUROPLASTICITY

How would you like to live in a city where every citizen can access resources that enhance their brain health, from well-funded mental health services to educational programs that promote lifelong learning?

This vision is achievable and essential for fostering a society that values cognitive health. Government initiatives are crucial in supporting neuroplasticity by funding mental health resources and launching public health campaigns focused on brain health. For instance, allocating funds to mental health clinics allows for providing therapies and treatments that promote neuroplasticity, such as cognitive behavioral therapy and mindfulness-based stress reduction programs. Public health campaigns can raise awareness about the importance of brain health, encouraging individuals to adopt habits that support neuroplasticity, such as regular exercise, a balanced diet, and adequate sleep. By prioritizing these initiatives, governments can create an environment where brain health is accessible, leading to a healthier, more resilient population.

Urban planning is another critical area where public policy can notably impact neuroplasticity. The design of cities and communities plays a vital role in promoting physical activity, social interactions, and mental wellness—key components of brain health. Features like sidewalks, bike lanes, and pedestrian-friendly infrastructure in walkable cities encourage regular physical exercise, enriching neuroplasticity. Accessible parks and green spaces provide opportunities for relaxation, socializing, and nature exposure, all of which contribute to improved cognitive functions and emotional health. Community recreational facilities, such as sports and cultural venues, provide spaces for people to engage in activities that stimulate their brain and foster social connections. By incorporating these elements into urban planning, policymakers can create environments that naturally support neuroplasticity and enhance the quality of life for residents.

Educational policies also play a pivotal role in promoting neuroplasticity from an early age. Early childhood education is critical for brain development, as the first few years of life are a period of rapid neural growth and plasticity. Policies that ensure access to high-quality early childhood education programs can provide children with the cognitive stimulation they need to develop powerful neural connections. These programs should incorporate activities that promote brain health, such as play-based learning, music, and language exposure. Ongoing adult education is equally important, as the brain remains plastic throughout life. Policies that support adult education and lifelong learning programs can help individuals continue to develop their cognitive abilities and adapt to new challenges. By fostering a culture of continuous learning, educational policies can support the brain's ability to grow and change at any age.

International examples of successful public policies highlight the potential impact of these initiatives. In Finland, the government has implemented educational policies emphasizing play-based learning and holistic development, resulting in high student engagement and academic achievement. The country's focus on early childhood education and lifelong learning has created a population that values education and cognitive health. Similarly, Singapore has invested in urban planning that prioritizes green spaces and walkability, creating a city where residents can easily engage in activities that support their brain health. The city's parks, gardens, and recreational facilities encourage physical activity and social interactions, contributing to overall healthier outcomes. These examples demonstrate how thoughtful public policies can create environments that naturally support neuroplasticity and enhance cognitive health.

In the United States, initiatives like the "Let's Move!" campaign have successfully promoted physical activity and healthy eating, which are crucial for brain health. By raising awareness and providing resources for individuals to make healthier choices, this campaign has improved physical and cognitive health across the country. Similarly, public health campaigns that focus on mental health awareness, such as the "Mental Health First Aid" program, provide education and resources for individuals to recognize and address mental health issues. These initiatives support individual brain health and contribute to a more informed and compassionate society.

Analyzing these successful policies demonstrates that government initiatives can play a crucial role in supporting neuroplasticity and cognitive health. Funding mental health resources, implementing urban planning that promotes physical activity and social interactions, and shaping educational policies to support continuous learning are all strategies that can foster environments conducive to brain health. As we continue to explore and understand the principles of neuroplasticity, the potential for public policy to enhance cognitive well-being becomes increasingly clear. Through thoughtful and intentional policies, governments can create a society where brain health is a priority, leading to a more resilient, adaptable, and thriving population.

6.5 TEST YOUR KNOWLEDGE

You sit comfortably with a cup of tea, reflecting on everything you've learned about creating a neuroplastic-friendly environment. You've explored how to design spaces that support brain health, the importance of social interactions, evolving educational approaches, corporate wellness programs, and the role of public policy. It's time to solidify your understanding and ensure you can apply these principles daily.

Question 1:True or False: Natural lighting is crucial for maintaining a healthy sleep-wake cycle and boosting cognitive functions.

Question 2: Multiple Choice: Which element is NOT typically considered when designing a neuroplastic-friendly environment?

A) Natural lighting
B) Noise control
C) Type of flooring
D) Nature integration

Question 3: True or False: Loneliness and social isolation can lead to structural changes in the brain, negatively affecting neuroplasticity.

Question 4: Multiple Choice: Which activity is most beneficial for enhancing social interactions and supporting brain health?

A) Watching TV alone
B) Joining a local club
C) Shopping online
D) Reading a book in isolation

Question 5: True or False: Flipped classrooms and project-based learning are innovative teaching methods that can enhance neuroplasticity in students.

Question 6: Multiple Choice: What is a key benefit of lifelong learning programs?

A) They only benefit young students
B) They promote continuous brain training throughout life
C) They are only useful for professional development
D) They have no impact on brain health

Question 7: True or False: Corporate wellness programs that include mindfulness sessions and stress management workshops can improve both employee well-being and productivity.

Question 8: Multiple Choice: What is a common strategy for implementing effective neuroplasticity-promoting wellness programs in the workplace?

A) Ignoring employee feedback
B) Offering a variety of program options
C) Mandating participation in all programs
D) Limiting the programs to senior management

Question 9: True or False: Urban planning that includes walkable cities and accessible parks can promote physical activity and enhance neuroplasticity.

Question 10: Multiple Choice: Which public policy initiative can support neuroplasticity from an early age?

A) Reducing funding for early childhood education
B) Ensuring access to high-quality early childhood
   education programs
C) Limiting adult education opportunities
D) Cutting mental health resources

Answers:

1. True
2. C) Type of flooring
3. True
4. B) Joining a local club
5. True
6. B) They promote continuous brain training throughout life
7. True
8. B) Offering a variety of program options
9. True
10. B) Ensuring access to high-quality early childhood education programs

Reflecting on these questions helps ensure that you understand the concepts covered in this chapter. Each principle, from the design of your living space to the policies shaping our communities, contributes to a broader understanding of nurturing and enhancing your brain's plasticity. Integrating these strategies into your daily life reinforces your knowledge and actively supports your mental health.

In the next chapter, we will explore personal stories of transformation, illustrating the real-life impact of neuroplasticity. These stories will provide inspiration and practical insights, showing how individuals have successfully applied neuroplastic principles to overcome challenges. Stay tuned for a closer look at the power of neuroplasticity in action.

CHAPTER SEVEN

PERSONAL STORIES OF TRANSFORMATION

Have you ever wondered what it feels like to face an impossible challenge and overcome it against all odds? Picture Tom, an active 55-year-old man who loved jogging and playing tennis. One ordinary morning, he woke up feeling different —his right side was numb, and his speech was slurred. Within hours, Tom's life took a drastic turn as he was diagnosed with a stroke. The initial prognosis was grim: doctors told him he might never speak clearly or walk unaided again. This chapter delves into Tom's incredible recovery journey, illustrating the transformative power of neuroplasticity.

7.1 STROKE SURVIVOR: A JOURNEY OF RECOVERY

Tom's initial challenges were staggering. The stroke severely affected the left hemisphere of his brain, which controls language and motor skills on the right side of the body. This resulted in apha-sia, a condition impairing his ability to communicate, and hemiplegia, causing paralysis on his right side. Everyday activities that once seemed trivial, like holding a fork or forming a sentence, became Herculean tasks. The traditional recovery expectations were modest: incremental improvements over years, with no guarantee of regaining full function. Yet, Tom was determined to defy these odds.

Tom's path to recovery hinged on neuroplasticity, the brain's remarkable ability to reorganize and form new neural connections. His rehabilitation began with constraint-induced movement therapy (CIMT). This technique involves restricting the use of the unaffected limb to force the brain to rewire itself to improve function in the affected limb. Tom's left arm was immobilized for hours each day, compelling him to use his right arm for tasks like brushing his teeth or picking up objects. This repetitive practice helped activate neuroplastic changes, gradually improving motor skills and strength in his right arm.

In addition to CIMT, cognitive rehabilitation exercises played a crucial role in Tom's recovery. Speech therapists introduced exercises designed to rebuild neural pathways for language. These included naming objects, forming sentences, and practicing conversations. Slowly but surely, Tom began to regain his ability to speak. He also engaged in intensive physical therapy, focusing on regaining mobility. Therapists utilized gait training exercises involving repetitive walking practice on a treadmill with body weight support, helping Tom relearn walking mechanics and enhancing his balance and coordination.

Tom's rehabilitation was also reinforced by activities designed to promote brain-derived neurotrophic factor (BDNF) production. As mentioned earlier, BDNF is a protein that supports the survival of existing neurons and encourages the growth of new neurons and synapses. Aerobic exercises, such as stationary cycling and swimming, were included in his regimen to boost BDNF levels. Additionally, a diet rich in polyphenols and omega-3 fatty acids was recommended, with foods like blueberries, salmon, and walnuts becoming staples to support his brain health.

Interactive Element: Reflection on Rehabilitation Progress

Take a moment to reflect on the types of challenges you might face in your daily life. Consider how you would apply the principles of neuroplasticity to overcome them. Would you use repetitive practice to improve a skill? Or incorporate physical exercise and a brain-healthy diet to enhance cognitive function. Write down three ways you can integrate neuroplastic techniques into your routine to address specific challenges you encounter.

Tom's journey was far from linear, with setbacks and moments of frustration, but his relentless dedication to his rehabilitation exercises paid off. Over the months, he began to see significant improvements. While not entirely fluent, his speech became intelligible enough for meaningful conversations. He regained enough strength and coordination in his right leg to walk short distances with a cane. These milestones were both physical and emotional triumphs, restoring his confidence and independence.

The power of Tom's story lies in its validation of neuroplasticity's potential. Through a combination of constraint-induced movement therapy, cognitive rehabilitation exercises, aerobic activities, and a brain-healthy diet, Tom's brain was able to rewire itself to compensate for the damage caused by the stroke. His journey underscores the importance of a holistic approach to recovery, integrating various techniques to promote neuroplastic changes. Tom's experience is a testament to the resilience of the human spirit and the brain's extraordinary capacity for adaptation and healing.

7.2 OVERCOMING LEARNING DISABILITIES THROUGH NEUROPLASTICITY

Consider Mia, a ten-year-old with a vibrant curiosity, yet facing substantial hurdles in her academic journey. Living with dyslexia, the tasks of reading and writing felt impossible for her. The letters on the page appeared scrambled, rendering comprehension a formidable challenge. Observing her peers easily navigate assignments demanding hours of effort only intensified her frustration. Misunderstood by teachers who perceived her efforts as lacking, Mia was trapped in a cycle of diminishing self-esteem and academic setbacks. Her school days were overshadowed by these continuous struggles, making each learning opportunity feel like a steep climb.

Mia's parents decided to seek specialized help and discovered neuroplastic-based interventions tailored to her needs. At the heart of Mia's intervention was brain training designed to target her specific cognitive deficits. One such method involved phonemic awareness exercises, which focused on helping Mia recognize and manipulate the sounds in words. These repetitive and intensive exercises engaged her brain to form new neural pathways that made decoding words easier. Adaptive learning technologies played a crucial role, with apps designed for dyslexic children offering interactive and engaging ways to practice reading. These apps used visual and auditory cues to reinforce learning, helping Mia bridge gaps in her phonological processing abilities.

These neuroplastic interventions marked the turning point in Mia's educational journey. One meaningful moment came when Mia's tutor introduced a multi-sensory reading program. This program combined visual, auditory, and kinesthetic learning strategies, allowing her to use her strengths to compensate for her weaknesses. For instance, tracing letters in the sand while saying the sounds out loud helped solidify her understanding in a way traditional methods hadn't. Another pivotal moment came when Mia began using a text-to-speech software that read aloud her school assignments. This tool improved her comprehension and allowed her to participate more meaningfully in classroom discussions, boosting her confidence.

As Mia continued with these interventions, her progress became apparent. She transitioned from reading simple sentences to tackling entire paragraphs with less struggle. Her writing improved as well, with notable clearer structure and fewer errors. These achievements were celebrated as academic milestones and personal victories that reshaped Mia's relationship with learning. The once-daunting task of reading became a source of pride, and her self-esteem flourished. Mia's newfound abilities opened doors that had previously seemed closed, and her academic performance soared.

In the long term, Mia's enhanced neuroplastic capabilities led to momentous achievements. She graduated from high school with honors —a feat once thought out of reach. Her newfound confidence in her abilities drove her to pursue higher education, enrolling in a college program focused on special education. Her experiences and the desire to help others facing similar challenges inspired her. Mia's academic success continued. She went on to earn a master's degree, specializing in educational psychology. Today, she's a passionate advocate for children with learning disabilities, working as a special education teacher.

Mia's story is a testament to the power of neuroplasticity and targeted interventions. By leveraging specialized tutoring and adaptive technologies, she was able to rewire her brain and overcome the limitations imposed by dyslexia. Her journey highlights the transformative potential of neuroplasticity, turning obstacles into opportunities and struggles into strengths. Through her experiences, Mia has achieved personal success and become a ray of hope and support for other children navigating similar paths.

Reflection Section: Identifying Personal Strengths and Weaknesses

Take a moment to think about a challenge you or someone you know faces. Write down three specific areas where improvement is needed. Next, identify three strengths that can be leveraged to address these areas. How can you apply neuroplastic principles, such as repetitive practice or multi-sensory learning, to overcome these challenges? Consider integrating adaptive technologies or specialized tutoring if applicable. Reflect on how these strategies might transform the educational or personal landscape, paving the way for long-term success.

Mia's achievements are not just about academic success but the broader impact of understanding and utilizing neuroplasticity. Her journey from struggling with dyslexia to becoming an advocate for special education illustrates the life-altering changes that targeted interventions can bring. Mia rewrote her story by focusing on her unique needs and strengths, demonstrating that learning disabilities can be managed and overcome with the correct approaches.

7.3 THE ROLE OF NEUROPLASTICITY IN CONQUERING ADDICTION

Rebecca's story is one of a vibrant woman whose life began to spiral out of control due to alcohol addiction. At first, it was just a glass of wine to unwind after work, but over time, it escalated to a bottle a night, then multiple bottles. Her addiction wasn't just a bad habit; it was deeply rooted in her brain's chemistry. Alcohol had hijacked her brain's reward system, flooding it with dopamine and creating powerful neural pathways that reinforced the addictive behavior. Every time she drank, those pathways strengthened, making it increasingly difficult to break the cycle. The neurological basis of addiction is complex, involving alterations in neurotransmitter activity and changes in brain circuitry, particularly in areas associated with reward, motivation, and self-control. Rebecca's battle with addiction was not only against the substance but also against the deeply ingrained neural patterns that perpetuated her dependence.

Rebecca's path to recovery involved neuroplasticity-based treatments designed to rewire her brain and break the cycle of addiction. Cognitive-behavioral therapy (CBT) was a cornerstone of her treatment. CBT helped Rebecca identify and challenge the negative thought patterns and behaviors that fueled her addiction. By recognizing these patterns, she could replace them with healthier, more constructive thoughts. This process was like pruning a garden: removing the weeds of negative thinking to allow the flowers of positive habits to grow. Another crucial component was mindfulness-based relapse prevention. Through mindfulness practices, Rebecca learned to stay present and observe her cravings without acting on them. This technique helped her develop a new relationship with her thoughts and feelings, reducing the power of her cravings and allowing her to respond more thoughtfully rather than react impulsively.

Key milestones marked Rebecca's recovery journey, each underscoring the pivotal role of neuroplasticity. Initially, even the thought of resisting a drink seemed impossible. Yet, through consistent application of CBT and mindfulness, she began to notice subtle shifts. One of the first milestones was her ability to go through an entire evening without drinking, using deep breathing and mindfulness techniques to cope with her cravings. This success was more than just a victory over alcohol; it was evidence of her brain's ability to form new and healthier neural pathways. As weeks turned into months, Rebecca's progress became increasingly evident. She started engaging in activities she had long abandoned, like painting and hiking, which provided joy and reinforced her positive neural connections.

Sustained change, however, required ongoing strategies to maintain sobriety and support neuroplasticity. Rebecca adopted a holistic approach, integrating lifestyle changes and continuous mental health support. Regular physical exercise became a staple in her routine, boosting her mood and brain health. Aerobic activities like jogging and cycling increase the production of BDNF, a protein that supports the growth of new neurons and strengthens existing ones. A balanced diet rich in omega-3 fatty acids, antioxidants, and vitamins further supported her brain's health and resilience. Rebecca also committed to regular mindfulness practice, setting aside time each day for meditation and reflection. These practices helped her stay attuned to her thoughts and feelings, allowing her to address any emerging cravings before they could take hold.

Continuous mental health support played a central role in Rebecca's sustained recovery. She attended weekly therapy sessions, which provided a space to discuss her challenges and successes and to refine her coping strategies. Support groups offered a sense of community and shared understanding, reinforcing her commitment to sobriety. Rebecca also found that educating herself about the science of neuroplasticity empowered her to stay motivated. Understanding that her brain was continuously adapting and evolving gave her hope and a sense of agency over her recovery.

Through the combined efforts of CBT, mindfulness, physical exercise, a nutritious diet, and ongoing mental health support, Rebecca's brain gradually rewired itself, allowing her to break free from the grip of addiction. Her story illustrates the impact of neuroplasticity in conquering addiction, transforming deeply ingrained behaviors, and fostering a healthier, more fulfilling life.

7.4 SENIORS IMPROVING MEMORY AND COGNITIVE FUNCTIONS

Let's shift our gears to Margaret, a lively woman in her seventies who once thrived on social engagements and intellectual pursuits. Over the past few years, she noticed her memory slipping. She struggled to recall names and frequently misplaced items and found it more challenging to follow conversations. These experiences were unsettling, not just because of the inconvenience but because they chipped away at her confidence. The initial cognitive decline affected her daily life drastically. Simple tasks like grocery shopping became daunting, and her once-active social life dwindled as she feared embarrassment from her memory lapses.

Seeing her growing frustration, Margaret's family sought ways to support her, leading them to explore neuroplastic interventions designed to boost cognitive functions. One of the first steps was enrolling her in a memory training program. These programs incorporated exercises targeting various aspects of memory, such as recall, recognition, and association. Margaret started with simple tasks like matching pictures and gradually advanced to more complex activities, such as remembering grocery lists and recounting stories. These exercises were designed to stimulate her brain and promote the formation of new neural connections.

Physical exercise also played a necessary role in Margaret's cognitive improvement. Her regimen included daily walks and light strength training. Since physical activity is known to increase the production of BDNF, Margaret found that her morning walks boosted her mood and sharpened her mind, making her feel more alert and engaged throughout the day.

Social engagement activities further enriched Margaret's neuroplastic interventions. Recognizing the importance of staying socially active, she joined a local book club and regularly attended community events. These interactions provided her with cognitive stimulation and emotional support, creating a positive feedback loop that enhanced her overall well-being. Engaging in conversations, participating in group activities, and learning new things from her peers all contributed to keeping her mind active and engaged.

The improvements Margaret observed were remarkable. Her memory recall became more reliable, and she regained her confidence in social settings. She could remember names and faces better and follow conversations with ease. Her problem-solving abilities also saw a boost. Tasks that once felt overwhelming, like planning a family gathering or managing her finances, became manageable again. These cognitive gains improved her daily life, allowing her to reclaim her independence and fully enjoy her activities.

Margaret's quality of life saw substantial enhancements due to the neuroplastic interventions she adopted. Her improved memory and cognitive functions made her feel more connected to her loved ones and her community. She could engage in meaningful conversations without fearing forgetting and participate in activities that brought her joy. This newfound confidence led her to explore new hobbies and interests, further enriching her life. She took up painting, something she had always wanted to try but never had the time for. This artistic pursuit provided her with a creative outlet and another avenue for cognitive stimulation.

Margaret's story exemplifies the impact of targeted neuroplastic interventions on seniors experiencing cognitive decline. She enhanced her cognitive functions through memory training programs, physical exercise, and social engagement activities. These improvements boosted her mental abilities and transformed her quality of life, allowing her to live independently and confidently.

7.5 YOUNG ADULTS USING NEUROPLASTICITY TO ENHANCE ACADEMIC PERFORMANCE

Alex, a college student who struggled with academic challenges, always needed help concentrating during lectures and retaining new information. This was more than occasional forgetfulness; it was a persistent issue affecting his grades and self-esteem. He often found himself staring at his textbooks, unable to absorb the material, and feeling overwhelmed by the volume of information he needed to learn. The traditional methods of studying—highlighting, rereading, and cramming—seemed ineffective, leaving Alex frustrated and anxious about his academic future.

Determined to find a solution, Alex explored neuroplastic techniques to improve his cognitive abilities. One of the first techniques he applied was spaced repetition learning. Unlike cramming, spaced repetition involves reviewing information at increasing intervals over time. This method leverages the brain's ability to strengthen neural connections through repeated exposure, enhancing long-term retention. Alex used digital flashcard apps that implemented spaced repetition algorithms, allowing him to study more efficiently and retain information better.

In addition to spaced repetition, Alex incorporated multimodal learning strategies into his study routine, which involves engaging multiple senses to process information. For example, while studying biology, Alex read the textbook, watched related videos, and used interactive 3D models to visualize concepts. This approach activated different brain areas, creating a richer and more integrated understanding of the material. By combining visual, auditory, and kinesthetic learning methods, Alex found that he could grasp complex topics more easily and remember them longer.

Targeted cognitive exercises were another critical component of Alex's academic transformation. These exercises aimed to improve specific cognitive functions such as attention, memory, and problem-solving. Alex used brain training apps that offered games and challenges designed to enhance these skills. Activities like memory-matching games, pattern recognition tasks, and logic puzzles became a regular part of his routine. Over time, these exercises helped improve his focus and cognitive flexibility, making it easier for him to switch between tasks and manage the demands of his coursework.

The results of these neuroplastic enhancements were irrefutable, as Alex's academic performance improved significantly. He began to see higher grades on his assignments and exams, which boosted his confidence and motivation. One of his most notable achievements was acing a challenging biochemistry exam that he had previously failed. This accomplishment demonstrated the effectiveness of the techniques he had adopted and reinforced his belief in his ability to succeed academically. His professors noticed the improvement and commended his progress, recognizing his dedication and hard work.

With his newfound academic abilities, Alex's future aspirations grew bolder. He began to consider career paths that he had once dismissed as unattainable. Empowered by his improved cognitive skills, Alex decided to pursue a degree in biomedical engineering, a field that combines his interests in biology and technology. He also became involved in research projects, contributing to studies on brain-computer interfaces and neuroprosthetics. These opportunities allowed him to apply his knowledge in practical settings and further develop his skills.

The confidence that Alex gained from leveraging neuroplasticity extended beyond academics. He became more active in extracurricular activities, joining clubs and organizations aligned with his interests. He took on leadership roles, organizing events and mentoring younger students who faced similar academic challenges. Alex's experience with neuroplastic techniques gave him a unique perspective and the tools to help others navigate their educational difficulties.

Alex's story is a tribute to the power of neuroplasticity in overcoming academic challenges and unlocking true potential. Through spaced repetition learning, multimodal strategies, and targeted cognitive exercises, Alex transformed his academic performance and future aspirations. His journey highlights the importance of adopting diverse and effective study methods to enhance cognitive functions and achieve academic success.

7.6 A CAREGIVER'S TALE: SUPPORTING NEUROPLASTICITY IN LOVED ONES

Susan, a devoted caregiver, faced a life-altering challenge when her husband, Mark, was diagnosed with a degenerative neurological condition. The initial shock and the mounting difficulties seemed almost too much to bear. Observing Mark struggle with everyday tasks, which he previously accomplished with ease, was a source of deep heartache. Activities such as dressing or recalling a recent conversation turned into major hurdles. Amidst these trials, Susan found herself in a delicate balancing act—caring for Mark while trying to preserve her own mental and physical health. The stress of the situation was tangible, leading to exhaustion, anxiety, and periods of overwhelming sadness. The emotional burden of witnessing the decline of a loved one left Susan feeling isolated and burdened by an crushing sense of responsibility.

In her quest to find ways to help Mark, Susan stumbled upon the concept of neuroplasticity. Intrigued by the idea that the brain could rewire itself, she began delving deeper into how these principles could support Mark's condition. Susan learned that neuroplasticity could be activated through specific exercises and lifestyle changes. She started with simple activities designed to stimulate Mark's brain. These included memory games, puzzles, and tasks that required fine motor skills. Each day, Susan would set aside time to engage Mark in these activities, ensuring they were both challenging and enjoyable. She also incorporated physical exercise into their routine, understanding that movement could promote the growth of new neurons. They began taking short walks together, gradually increasing the distance as Mark's strength improved.

One of the most significant changes Susan made was in their diet. She learned that certain foods could support brain health and enhance neuroplasticity. Susan started preparing meals rich in omega-3 fatty acids, antioxidants, and other brain-boosting nutrients. She included fish, berries, nuts, and leafy greens in their diet, hoping to provide the best environment for Mark's brain to adapt and grow. Additionally, Susan introduced mindfulness and relaxation techniques to help manage stress. They practiced deep breathing exercises and meditation, fostering a calm and focused mind for both of them.

As weeks turned into months, Susan observed noticeable improvements in Mark's condition. His memory improved, and he became more engaged in their daily activities. Tasks that had previously seemed impossible were now within reach. Mark's coordination and motor skills also showed signs of enhancement, allowing him to regain some of his independence. These changes were not just physical but emotional triumphs, reigniting a sense of hope and possibility. Susan's dedication and the neuroplastic techniques she implemented had an overpowering impact, demonstrating the brain's remarkable ability to adapt and heal.

Encouraged by the progress, Susan felt compelled to share her newfound knowledge with others in similar situations. She joined online forums and local support groups, eager to connect with other caregivers facing the same challenges. Susan's story resonated with many, offering hope and practical advice. She began organizing workshops and meetings, sharing the neuroplastic techniques that had worked for Mark. These gatherings became a source of strength and inspiration for the caregiving community, fostering a sense of solidarity and shared purpose.

Through her efforts, Susan helped create a supportive community that embraced the principles of neuroplasticity in caregiving. Caregivers exchanged tips, shared successes, and supported each other through setbacks. Susan's experience underscored the importance of education and community in caregiving. By understanding and applying neuroplastic concepts, caregivers could make meaningful differences in the lives of their loved ones. The ripple effect of Susan's journey extended far beyond her household, touching countless lives and reaffirming the power of resilience, knowledge, and compassion.

7.7 TEST YOUR KNOWLEDGE

You've read about the extraordinary transformations driven by the power of neuroplasticity. These stories showcase how the brain's ability to rewire can significantly improve various aspects of life, from overcoming learning disabilities to conquering addiction. Now, it's time to reflect on what you've learned and ensure you can apply these principles in your daily life.

The following quiz will reinforce critical concepts and practical applications of neuroplasticity. Take your time with each question and consider how the information you've gathered can translate into tangible actions for enhancing brain health and cognitive functions.

Question 1: True or False: Neuroplasticity allows the brain to create new pathways and reorganize functions to compensate for tissue damage after a stroke.

Question 2: Multiple Choice: Which of the following is a key strategy to overcome learning disabilities through neuroplasticity?

    A) Medication
    B) Specialized tutoring with brain training techniques
    C) Ignoring the disability
    D) Traditional classroom methods

Question 3: True or False: Cognitive-behavioral therapy and mindfulness-based relapse prevention help rewire the brain to combat addiction.

Question 4: Multiple Choice: What role does brain-derived neurotrophic factor (BDNF) play in neuroplasticity?

A) It inhibits neural growth

B) It promotes the growth of new neurons and synapses

C) It has no effect on neurons

D) It decreases cognitive function

Question 5: True or False: Memory training programs and physical exercise can improve cognitive functions in seniors experiencing age-related decline.

Question 6: Multiple Choice: Which techniques effectively manage ADHD through neuroplasticity?

A) Positive reinforcement and structured routines

B) Sporadic and unplanned activities

C) Excessive screen time

D) High-sugar diets

Question 7: True or False: Spaced repetition learning involves reviewing information at increasing intervals to enhance long-term retention.

Question 8: Multiple Choice: Which physical activity is known to boost BDNF levels and enhance cognitive function?

A) Watching television

B) Aerobic exercises like jogging and cycling

C) Sitting for long periods

D) Sleeping excessively

Question 9: True or False: Adaptive learning technologies can help individuals with learning disabilities by providing interactive and engaging ways to practice essential skills.

Question 10: Multiple Choice: What is a common benefit observed in individuals who use neuroplastic techniques to overcome addiction?

A) Increased cravings

B) Development of new, healthy habits

C) Worsening of addiction

D) No change in behavior

Answers:

1. True
2. B) Specialized tutoring with brain training techniques
3. True
4. B) It promotes the growth of new neurons and synapses
5. True
6. A) Positive reinforcement and structured routines
7. True
8. B) Aerobic exercises like jogging and cycling
9. True
10. B) Development of new, healthy habits

These questions are designed to help you internalize the principles of neuroplasticity and understand their practical applications. Reflect on your responses and consider incorporating these strategies into your daily routine to enhance your brain's adaptability and functionality.

Neuroplasticity is a powerful tool that can transform lives, as demonstrated by the stories in this chapter. Whether overcoming a significant health challenge, improving cognitive abilities, or supporting a loved one, understanding and leveraging neuroplastic principles can lead to great changes. As you continue to explore the concept, remember that small, consistent efforts can lead to significant, lasting improvements in your cognitive health and overall well-being.

CONCLUSION

This book starts with Maria, the older woman whose remarkable recovery from a severe stroke introduced us to the concept of neuroplasticity. Thanks to the brain's incredible ability to reorganize itself, her journey was about regaining lost skills and discovering new passions and possibilities. Neuroplasticity is like the brain's personal trainer, constantly reshaping and strengthening its neural muscles to adapt to life's challenges. This concept is not just a scientific curiosity; it's a powerful tool that can reshape lives, including yours.

I can attest that neuroplasticity is reshaping my life.

Throughout this book, we've explored how neuroplasticity can help you recover from injuries, enhance learning, and maintain overall brain health. We've seen that the brain can adapt and thrive by forming new neural connections, even in the face of adversity. This ability to rewire makes neuroplasticity essential for a fulfilling and resilient life.

The importance of a neuroplastic-friendly lifestyle cannot be over-stated. Daily choices can create a "virtuous cycle" of brain health, where each positive action fuels another. For example, a nutritious diet provides the building blocks for neurotransmitters, enhancing sleep quality. Better sleep improves cognitive functioning, which helps manage stress, creating a ripple effect of wellness.

Here are the Top 5 Actions you can start applying today to boost your brain's neuroplasticity:

1. **Eat a Brain-Healthy Diet:** Incorporate omega-3 fatty acids, antioxidants, and vitamins. Think salmon, blueberries, and leafy greens.
2. **Exercise Regularly:** Aim for at least 30 minutes of aerobic activity, such as walking, jogging, or swimming, on most days of the week.
3. **Prioritize Sleep:** Ensure you get 7-9 hours of quality sleep every night and establish a consistent sleep schedule.
4. **Manage Stress:** Practice daily mindfulness, meditation, or deep breathing exercises.
5. **Stay Mentally Active:** Engage in intellectually stimulating activities such as puzzles, reading, and learning new skills.

These actions form the foundation of a lifestyle that supports neuro-plasticity, setting the stage for continuous brain growth and adapt-ability.

Practical applications of neuroplasticity are within your reach. Simple habits like starting your day with a 10-minute meditation, a brisk walk, and a brain-boosting breakfast can lead to significant cognitive improvements. Engage in brain training games, practice mindfulness, and work on overcoming negative thought patterns.

These small, consistent steps will help you incorporate neuroplastic principles into your daily life, making a tangible difference.

Remember, neuroplasticity is a lifelong process. Whether you're a child learning to read or a senior looking to maintain cognitive health, the brain's capacity for change never diminishes. Inspiring examples in this book, like Margaret, who improved her memory and independence in her seventies, show there is always time to start. "The brain never stops growing as long as we keep challenging it," says Dr. Michael Merzenich, a pioneer in the field of neuroplasticity.

The personal transformation stories we've shared highlight the universal potential for change. From Tom's stroke recovery to Mia overcoming dyslexia, Rebecca conquering addiction, and Alex enhancing his academic performance, these narratives are testaments to the power of neuroplasticity. These stories are inspiring and practical, offering real-life applications you can adopt.

Creating a supportive environment is paramount, so design your living and working spaces to promote mental wellness. Incorporate natural light, control noise, and bring in elements of nature. Commit to making one change in your environment—maybe add a plant to your workspace or set up a quiet reading nook. Share your progress with friends and family or on social media to foster a community of support.

Now, it's time for action. Embrace a neuroplastic lifestyle by applying the principles and techniques outlined in this book. Set a goal right now: Which neuroplasticity technique will you incorporate into your daily routine first? Write it down, schedule it, and start today. Remember, your brain's potential is limitless but requires active participation.

Thank you for joining me on this journey of understanding and applying neuroplasticity. Committing to enhancing your brain's plasticity is a step towards a healthier, more fulfilled life. For continued learning and support, consider exploring recommended readings like "The Brain That Changes Itself" by Norman Doidge, websites like BrainHQ, and apps like Lumosity.

As we conclude, I leave you with a message of hope and empowerment: Your brain is not a fixed entity—it's a dynamic, evolving masterpiece. Embrace this journey with curiosity and courage, and watch your life transform. Challenges are growth opportunities, and you can turn those challenges into triumphs with neuroplasticity. Your brain, your life, your potential—endlessly adaptable, always growing.

REFERENCES

Cherry, K. (2023, August 14). *Neuroplasticity: How experience changes the brain.* Verywell Mind. https://www.verywellmind.com/what-is-brain-plasticity-2794886

Bavelier, D., & Neville, H. J. (2002). *Adult neuroplasticity: More than 40 years of research.* Progress in Brain Research, 138, 125-133. https://www.ncbi.nlm.nih.gov/pmc/articles/PMC4026979/

Hölzel, B. K., Ott, U., Gard, T., Hempel, H., Weygandt, M., Morgen, K., & Vaitl, D. (2008). *The effect of meditation on brain structure: Cortical thickness mapping.* NeuroReport, 19(10), 1049-1053. https://www.ncbi.nlm.nih.gov/pmc/articles/PMC3541490/

Sossin, W. S., Lacaille, J. C., Castellucci, V. F., & Belleville, S. (2005). *Neurotransmitter roles in synaptic modulation, plasticity, and learning in the nervous system.* Progress in Brain Research, 147, 121-130. https://www.ncbi.nlm.nih.gov/pmc/articles/PMC2849868/

National Institute on Aging. (2023, July 17). *MIND and Mediterranean diets linked to fewer signs of Alzheimer's brain pathology.* https://www.nia.nih.gov/news/mind-and-mediterranean-diets-linked-fewer-signs-alzheimers-brain-pathology

Davis, B. N., Pilch, M., Wojtyna, S. C., Mahon, M., Kolman, P., MacDougall, H., ... & Brosnan, M. J. (2022). *Effects of strength training on BDNF in healthy young adults.* Journal of Strength and Conditioning Research, 36(5), 1450-1456. https://www.ncbi.nlm.nih.gov/pmc/articles/PMC9658702/

Stickgold, R., & Walker, M. P. (2005). *The role of sleep in memory consolidation.* Journal of Sleep Research, 14(1), 49-59. https://www.ncbi.nlm.nih.gov/pmc/articles/PMC10728269/

Singh, S., Sharma, P., & Chopra, M. (2021). *Chronic stress induces significant gene expression changes in rat brain regions.* Neurobiology of Stress, 14, 100321. https://www.ncbi.nlm.nih.gov/pmc/articles/PMC7850288/

Kim, K. (2022, June 7). *This neuroscientist-approved morning routine is great for peak brain health.* The Optimist Daily. https://www.optimistdaily.com/2022/06/do-this-in-the-morning-for-peak-brain-health-according-to-neuroscientists/

Wynn, S. (2022, April 14). *Do brain-training apps really work?* Discover Magazine. https://www.discovermagazine.com/mind/do-brain-training-apps-really-work

Mayo Clinic Staff. (2023, May 13). *Memory loss: 7 tips to improve your memory.* Mayo Clinic. https://www.mayoclinic.org/healthy-lifestyle/healthy-aging/in-depth/memory-loss/art-20046518

Chernoff, M. (2021, May 5). *Cognitive restructuring: Techniques and examples.* Healthline. https://www.healthline.com/health/cognitive-restructuring

Big Life Journal. (2022, July 8). *Teaching kids about the brain: Neuroplasticity activities.* https://biglifejournal.com/blogs/blog/teach-kids-growth-mindset-neuro plasticity-activities

Kays, J. L., Hurley, R. A., & Taber, K. H. (2012). *The power of connection: Social engagement and mental health.* Aging True. https://agingtrue.org/the-power-of-connection-social-engagement-and-mental-health/

Carstensen, L. L., & Pasupathi, M. (2003). *Intergenerational learning: Proven benefits for both elders and youth.* Center on Reinventing Public Education. https://crpe.org/intergenerational-learning/

Lindauer, R. J., & Rosenfeld, J. P. (2015). *Neuroplasticity in response to cognitive behavior therapy for depression: A systematic review of fMRI studies.* Translational Psychiatry, 5(1), e578. https://www.nature.com/articles/tp2015218

Walsh, B. (2011, January 21). *Eight weeks to a better brain.* Harvard Gazette. https://news.harvard.edu/gazette/story/2011/01/eight-weeks-to-a-better-brain/

Smith, M. (2023, June 10). *Biofeedback therapy: Uses and benefits.* WebMD. https://www.webmd.com/pain-management/biofeedback-therapy-uses-benefits

Halperin, J. M., & Healey, D. M. (2011). *Physical exercise in attention deficit hyperactivity disorder: Impacts and mechanisms.* Journal of Child Psychology and Psychiatry, 52(9), 803-813. https://www.ncbi.nlm.nih.gov/pmc/arti cles/PMC6945516/

Lee, A. Y. (2023). *Designing for human wellbeing: The integration of architecture and psychology.* Frontiers of Architectural Research, 12(4), 567-581. https://www.sciencedirect.com/science/article/pii/S2090447922004130

Bremner, J. D., & Vermetten, E. (2001). *Social influences on neuroplasticity: Stress and interventions.* Dialogues in Clinical Neuroscience, 3(2), 197-205. https://www.ncbi.nlm.nih.gov/pmc/articles/PMC3491815/

Boss, S. (2014, October 21). *Neuroplasticity: Learning physically changes the brain.* Edutopia. https://www.edutopia.org/neuroscience-brain-based-learning-neuroplas ticity

American Chamber of Commerce Hong Kong. (2022, March 9). *Neuroplasticity, workplace wellness & employee productivity.* https://amchamhk.glueup.com/en/ event/neuroplasticity-workplace-wellness-employee-productivity-14041/

Flint Rehab. (2023, February 28). *Neuroplasticity after stroke: How the brain overcomes injury.* https://www.flintrehab.com/neuroplasticity-after-stroke/

Cajal Academy. (2022, September 15). *Addressing learning disabilities through neuroplasticity interventions.* https://www.cajalacademy.org/academics/neuroplas ticity-interventions/

Cumberland Heights. (2022, October 7). *Neuroplasticity and recovery: How your brain heals*. https://www.cumberlandheights.org/blogs/neuroplasticity-for-recovery/

WE'D LOVE YOUR FEEDBACK!

Dear Reader,

Thank you for choosing *Neuroplasticity for Beginners* as your guide on this transformative journey. I sincerely hope the insights shared in this book have helped you better understand the brain's amazing capacity to adapt and change.

If this book has inspired you, deepened your curiosity, or answered your neuroplasticity questions, I'd be grateful if you could take a moment to leave a review. Your honest feedback helps me grow as an author and helps others discover the benefits of understanding how our brains can rewire for positive change.

Why Your Review Matters

Reviews help other readers discover the book and understand how neuroplasticity can apply to their own lives. Whether it's a quick sentence or a more detailed reflection, your review is important in spreading the message of growth and personal empowerment.

How to Leave a Review

It's simple:

1. Head to the platform where you purchased the book, such as Amazon.
2. Find where you place orders (Returns & Orders is in the menu on Amazon).
3. Find your order of *Neuroplasticity for Beginners* and choose Write a Product Review.

What to Include in Your Review

If you're not sure what to say, consider these questions:

- What did you find most helpful or eye-opening about neuroplasticity?
- Did this book change how you think about your brain's potential?
- Were the examples and explanations easy to understand for a beginner?

Your feedback, in any form, is appreciated!

Thank you once again for reading. I'm thrilled that you've taken this first step toward understanding and harnessing the power of your brain.

With gratitude,

   - Hector J. Bordas, Author of *Neuroplasticity for Beginners*

ABOUT THE AUTHOR

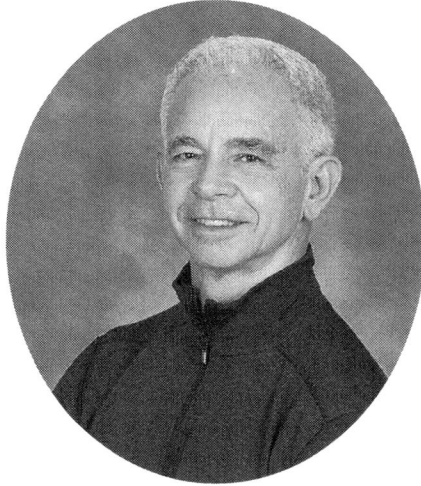

With over 25 years of leadership and team-building experience, Hector J Bordas has a knack for helping individuals and organizations unlock their full potential. His career spans from leading large-scale public works projects in Los Angeles County to founding national initiatives that address renewable energy challenges. Known for his ability to break down silos, foster collaboration, and drive cultural change, Hector has worked with diverse teams across engineering, environmental planning, and political strategy.

In his work, Hector challenges leaders to think critically, act decisively, and build a results-driven culture. Whether transforming teams of engineers or uniting water resource agencies, he's all about creating lasting impact through practical, actionable steps. His passion for personal growth and development, particularly through the lens of neuroplasticity, inspired him to write *Neuroplasticity for Beginners*, where he simplifies the science of the brain's adaptability for readers looking to harness its power for self-improvement.

When Hector isn't coaching leaders or speaking on team dynamics, you can find him exploring new ways to blend science and strategy to tackle today's most complex challenges.

Made in the USA
Middletown, DE
06 April 2025